Kinesiology

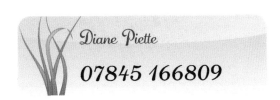
Diane Piette
07845 166809

ISBN: 978-0-9542439-7-5

Published by:

Life-Work Potential Limited
Sea View House
Long Rock
Penzance
Cornwall
TR20 8JF
England

Tel: + 44 (0)1736 719030
www.lifeworkpotential.com

Kinesiology

Jane Thurnell-Read

Other books by the author:

Verbal Questioning Skills For Kinesiologists
ISBN: 978-0-9542439-1-3, Life-Work Potential, 2004

Energy Mismatch
ISBN: 978-0-9542439-3-7, Life-Work Potential, 2004

Allergy A To Z
ISBN: 978-0-9542439-2-0, Life-Work Potential, 2005

Geopathic Stress
ISBN: 978-0-9542439-4-4 Life-Work Potential, 2006

Health Kinesiology: The Muscle Testing System That Talks To The Body
ISBN 978-0-9542439-6-8, Life-Work Potential Limited, 2009

Nutritional Testing For Kinesiologists And Dowsers
ISBN: 978-0-9542439-5-1, Life-Work Potential Limited, 2009

Writing a book and seeing it published is never a lone enterprise, although the name on the cover is of just one person – me.

There are many people who have contributed to this book without knowing it over the twenty plus years I have been involved in kinesiology. I have learnt from people who have taught me, from conference speakers, from books and journals I have read, from people I have met at workshops and conferences, from the students I have taught and, of course, from the many clients I have seen.

There are also people who have helped me specifically with this project. Many of them are mentioned by name in the book, but I'd also like to mention here Joyce Couper and Terry Larder, who have helped broaden my knowledge and understanding of the kinesiology systems I have not been exposed to myself. When I was unsure, I was able to check with them the accuracy of some of the things I wanted to say.

My partner, John Payne, has supported me throughout the process and has read and re-read the manuscript many times, reducing my errors and adding to the clarity of what I have written. Discussion with him about concepts and procedures, as ever, has been valuable and thought-provoking.

I hope this book will help promote kinesiology as a therapy that can totally change people's lives. It has done this for me.

I do not cover every kinesiology system in this book, but omission should not be taken to imply that a particular kinesiology system is unimportant or without value. From my own training I know more about some kinesiologies than others. For those I know less about I have had to rely on studying training manuals and/or talking to teachers and practitioners. Some kinesiology systems seem to have an abundance of people who wanted to communicate with me and help me understand about their kinesiology, whereas for others I found it difficult to make any useful contacts.

Legislation varies from country to country on the health claims practitioners are allowed to make. Claims of therapeutic benefits that are considered legitimate in one country may not be allowed in another. In addition, due to legislative changes a claim or comment made at the time the client was seen might now be deemed illegal.

Contents

Introduction

Let me first tell you how to pronounce it. It is kin-easy-ology, although a few people pronounce it kine-easy-ology. There are many different kinesiology systems, but they all use the same basic tool - muscle testing, also called muscle monitoring.

The word kinesiology means 'the study of movement' and was originally used to describe a field of medicine concerned with the working of joints and muscles. There are still people known as kinesiologists who work in conventional medicine, particularly in North America.

Since the 1960's, other systems of kinesiology have evolved from it, based on the work and insights of an American chiropractor, Dr George Goodheart. These are the therapies we will be looking at in this book.

Muscle testing is a painless procedure involving the practitioner applying gentle pressure to specific parts of the body (often arms and legs) to test the response of the underlying muscle. The particular part of the body involved is placed in a specific position in order, as far as possible, to isolate the muscle that is being tested. The muscle will either easily be able to resist the pressure from the practitioner or will give way. The kinesiologist uses this response to access information about what is happening within the body and what is needed to improve health and wellbeing. (See page 14 for a more detailed explanation.)

This amazing tool was developed by George Goodheart into a system that became known as Applied Kinesiology. Subsequently John Thie took elements of it and developed a system called Touch for Health, which was designed for use by people without any formal medical training to use in their homes and with their families and friends in both a preventive and in a restorative way.

Over the years many people in many different countries have learnt Applied Kinesiology and/or Touch for Health. Some of them have gone on to develop their own kinesiology systems either for use by the general public or, more usually, by practitioners. (See page 46 onwards). They offer a wide variety of approaches and techniques but all share the same tool - muscle testing (muscle monitoring). Each kinesiology reflects the experience, knowledge and interest of its creator. All kinesiologies also share many basic concepts and techniques and many of these are covered in this book.

Kinesiology produces more than its fair share of miracles for a therapy that is so casually dismissed by some as being rubbish, bizarre, silly, and only of interest to the gullible and the desperate.

You will read about some amazing things in this book that cannot be explained by current scientific and medical knowledge. Some improvements in symptoms may happen anyway, some may happen because of the placebo effect (see page 44), but there are others that defy any conventional explanation: animals or children too young to understand what was happening or clients who were sceptical or had a rigid scientific background. Kinesiology has attracted practitioners and developers with rigorous scientific backgrounds including doctorates (PhDs) in solid state physics (Diego Vellam, see page 79), in physiological psychology (Jimmy Scott, see page 84), in geology (Wayne Topping, see page 173) and biology and physiology (Charles Krebs, see page 50) and a research scientist in molecular biology (Barbara Grimwade, see page 81). Susan Eardlcy has been awarded a doctorate by Southampton University (UK) for her work showing the effectiveness of one kinesiology system in the management of chronic low back pain (see page 136). People with a medical background have also become deeply involved and committed to kinesiology, including Bruce Dewe (see page 136), a medical doctor , and Helen Bradley (see page 164), a speech and language therapist.

I have been involved in kinesiology for more than twenty years and during that time I have often met people who have said something to me along the lines of: I'm a scientist so, of course, I can't accept this. What an unscientific attitude to dismiss something without investigation, assuming that it cannot be correct because it does not fit current understanding.

Some critics dismiss kinesiology and similar therapies, claiming it attracts the woolly-minded and will not stand up to real scrutiny. In fact, kinesiology attracts people who are prepared to assess what they see objectively and without preconceptions.

History/Origins Of Kinesiology

The originator of kinesiology muscle testing as we know it was a US chiropractor called George Goodheart. His work ultimately resulted in a system now known as Applied Kinesiology.

George Goodheart & Applied Kinesiology

I am indebted to an article on the history of kinesiology on the web site of the International College Of Applied Kinesiology (www.icak.com) for some of the information in this section.

Although Dr Goodheart is recognised as the founder of kinesiology as a therapeutic system, the original work in this field was done by an orthopaedic surgeon, R.W. Lovett, in the 1920's. He developed a system for testing and grading the functioning of muscles. This work was further developed and systematized by Henry and Florence Kendall, who published a book in 1949, entitled *Muscle Testing And Function*.

In the early 1960's George Goodheart developed this work further. His first major insight was into the relationship between back pain and weak muscles. At that time back pain was understood to occur as a result of muscle spasm. Treatment was, therefore, focussed on relaxing the tense muscle or muscles. Goodheart saw back pain occurring as a result of muscular weakness. In his view muscle weakness (or inhibition as it is known technically) results in an associated muscle becoming tight, resulting in pain. From this understanding it follows that the muscle that needs attention is the weak muscle, as the tight muscle is a response to, not a cause of, the problem. As the weak muscle is corrected, the tight muscle lets go of its tension.

Goodheart's next major insight came when he examined a patient who was unable to work because of shoulder instability. He observed nodules in the muscle insertion and he applied heavy pressure with his fingers to reduce these nodules. Immediately afterwards the man was able to move his shoulder in a way he had not been able to do for fifteen years. Goodheart checked other patients and found that many responded to this vigorous stimulation at either the origin or insertion of the weak muscle. At the time it was believed that this was correcting micro-tears in the muscle fibres. This procedure became known as the origin/insertion technique (see page 38).

Goodheart also found that particular symptoms were often related to weaknesses in particular muscles. He then amalgamated his research with the work done in the 1930's by Frank Chapman, an osteopath. Chapman had examined the bodies of patients hospitalised for a range of problems. He found that people often had tender nodules on their bodies. These nodules were in the same place for people with similar symptoms, although not necessarily in the physical area of the problem. Chapman discovered that if he massaged the tender places on the body, the area would stop being tender and people's health often improved. He believed that he had found an internal switch or switches for each organ of the body and that stimulation of these points lead to a draining of the organ via the lymph system.

3

Goodheart found that these lymphatic points related to muscles: a particularly tender set of nodules (mapped by Chapman as relating to a particular organ system) would also correspond with a particular weak muscle or muscles. Massaging the tender nodules lead to a strengthening of the muscle and an improvement in symptoms associated with that organ. These nodules subsequently became known as neurolymphatic points (see page 37).

Goodheart also used the work of Terence Bennett, a chiropractic physician. Working in the 1930's Bennett had identified pulse spots that, when activated, improved blood supply to specific organs of the body and enhanced their function. These points, which were mainly on the head, became known in kinesiology as neurovascular points (see page 37).

In the 1960's Goodheart published a paper entitled "Chinese Lessons for Modern Chiropractic". He had found that pressing on acupuncture points could bring about changes, and so he concluded that needles were not essential for obtaining a positive result.

By now Goodheart had identified different ways of strengthening weak muscles using:

- Origin/insertion massage
- Neuro lymphatic points
- Neuro vascular points
- Acupuncture points

Initially Goodheart had seen muscle weakness as a sign of injury within the muscle and that the origin/insertion massage was correcting this. Gradually he had come to realise that muscle weakness could be an indicator of a less localised, more systemic problem. He had also discovered that using these muscle strengthening techniques often led to a corresponding improvement in the vitality and health of a body organ.

Goodheart understood that muscle testing could act as a language between the doctor and patient, and that if he worked to strengthen muscles, other health problems would improve or even disappear. This series of insights really opened up the depth and breadth of his work.

Goodheart then turned his attention to nutrition. He found that some foods and vitamin supplements would consistently strengthen particular muscles, so he began carefully to record his findings. He also looked at the importance of cranial bones to the health of the body. Microscopic movement in these bones allows for the proper flow of cerebro-spinal fluid.

By 1968 he had a coherent system, giving him various techniques he could use to bring about better body functioning and improved health. Although he was having a lot of success at strengthening muscles, he often found it difficult in cases where bilateral muscles were involved. This is where the same muscle on both sides of the body tested weak. Eventually he found the problem was often vertebral fixation (restricted movement of groups of vertebral segments). Goodheart found a specific chiropractic adjustment would often be the key to relieving this problem. Goodheart went on to identify other procedures that could be safely used by chiropractic doctors.

In 1974 he had another major insight which resulted in a procedure that became known as therapy localisation (see page 31). He found that he could use an indicator muscle (see page 18) to find an area of the body that needed attention. The patient touched an area of their own body with their hand, while he tested any muscle. If the area touched needed therapy, the muscle would weaken (if it had previously tested strong) or strengthen (if it had previously tested weak). Goodheart also found that, once the correct therapy had been applied, there would no longer be a change in the muscle (from strong to weak or from weak to strong).

This can seem a little confusing: the chiropractor tests a muscle and finds it tests weak, applies a therapy and the muscle still tests weak. But here it is important to realise that the muscle is being used as an <u>indicator</u> and is not being tested for its own integrity as in all of Goodheart's earlier work.

Goodheart gave the name Applied Kinesiology (AK) to his system. In 1976 The International College of Applied Kinesiology (ICAK) was established to promote research and the teaching of applied kinesiology muscle testing.

The ICAK describes Applied Kinesiology in this way:

> … a system which evaluates the structural, chemical and mental aspects of a person, has attracted doctors from all fields of health care. It utilizes standard muscle testing, as well as other accepted methods of diagnosis. Nutrition, diet, manipulation, acupressure, exercise and education are used therapeutically to help restore well-being.

Before studying Applied Kinesiology, practitioners have training in other specialist health modalities such as medicine, osteopathy, chiropractic or dentistry, but not everyone in these professions is also an Applied Kinesiologist. People who satisfactorily complete the ICAK training are known as ICAK diplomates.

John Thie & Touch for Health

John Thie was also a US chiropractor and he trained with Goodheart, and they became personal friends. Thie wanted Goodheart to develop a kinesiology syllabus for non-chiropractors, one that could be used by chiropractic assistants, nurses and even lay people. Thie and his wife Carrie had for a long time had a desire to help families be healthier through natural methods. Thie kept encouraging Goodheart to write a book aimed at ordinary people and using some of the techniques from applied kinesiology on a self-help basis. In the end Goodheart told Thie to write the book himself. Thie realised that writing a book aimed at lay people needed a lot of thought. Meanwhile he and his wife started to run seminars in these techniques, and gradually participants came to them and said they would like to be able to teach the information to others.

While the book was being written, the Thies taught the first nine prospective teachers. Thie found additional help via his chiropractic practice. A patient of his, Mary Marks (a writer), Mary's mother, Pat Gill (an anatomical artist) and her husband, (a graphic artist) helped with various aspects of the book.

Originally the Thies called the system Health From Within, but (at Pat Gill's suggestion) changed the name to Touch for Health. The first book was printed in 1973 and was hugely successful, so was quickly reprinted.

John Thie had envisaged chiropractors using applied kinesiology and the public using Touch for Health coming together in a spirit of co-operation and harmony:

> I originally believed, as I helped to organize the ICAK and wrote the Touch for Health book for lay and paraprofessional use, that there would be one Kinesiology organization whose membership would include professionals from all medical specialties, paraprofessionals in the healing arts and lay teachers of the Touch for Health classes.
> (www.touch4health.com/history.html)

Thie organised seminars, but gradually the chiropractors stopped attending, and the members of the ICAK (International College of Applied Kinesiology) decided that membership of their organisation should be exclusively for professionals who were licensed to diagnose. This excluded many paraprofessionals and TFH lay teachers.

In 1975 the Touch for Health Foundation was established and the training programme expanded rapidly. Some of the people who learnt Touch for Health began to expand and systematise it in different ways, creating new modalities with new names.

Touch for Health continued to grow and teachers took the information to other countries, including Argentina, Australia, Brazil, Canada, Germany, Ireland, Japan, the Netherlands, New Zealand, South Africa, UK, Russia, Switzerland and the Ukraine. The TFH book was translated into Braille, Danish, Dutch, French, German, Italian, Japanese, Portuguese, Polish, Slovak, Russian Spanish and Swedish. TFH Associations were also set up in many countries to promote Touch for Health.

In 1990 the Touch for Health Foundation was closed, as John and Carrie Thie decided to step down from such active involvement in the promotion of TFH. The International Kinesiology College based in Zurich Switzerland took over the certification of TFH trainers.

Nevertheless John Thie continued to work and produce new insights and ideas. In 1992, for example, in the revised Touch for Health manual he described a new way of correcting bilateral muscle inhibition. Up to this time the most effective correction for this problem had been a chiropractic adjustment, which was unsuitable for non-chiropractors. Thie called the new procedure spinal reflex technique (see page 37.)

Touch for Health (see page 160) remains a system designed for people to use with family and friends, although some kinesiologists and other practitioners will use aspects of it in their practice.

Other Kinesiologies

Some of the people who attended Touch for Health classes went on to develop their own branch of kinesiology, taking the original concepts in different directions. Although Touch for Health itself was aimed at the general public, many of these new kinesiologies became oriented more to the professional practitioner seeing patients or clients. Over the years further kinesiologies have been developed building on aspects of different existing kinesiologies. There is more information on these different kinesiology systems starting on page 46. Some of the techniques and concepts from these different kinesiology systems have fed back into the basic Touch for Health teaching.

There are fundamental differences between Applied Kinesiology practitioners (ICAK diplomates) and other kinesiologists. Applied kinesiologists have formal medical training in chiropractic, osteopathy, dentistry, medicine, etc., whereas other practitioners may not have a medical or physical manipulation background. AK practitioners are licensed to diagnose and treat medical conditions, whereas most other kinesiologists work with imbalances and stress.

Confusingly some people use the term 'applied kinesiology' as an umbrella term for all kinesiologies, covering those such as ICAK members who are licensed to make a medical diagnosis and other practitioners who are not. The ICAK has legal rights to the trademark Professional Applied Kinesiology and the term PAK.

The word kinesiology itself is open to confusion, as it is also used to describe the regulated health profession that focuses on physical activity with a strong basis in science and medicine. This is particularly prominent in the USA.

Subtle Energy, Elements, Meridians & Muscles

In order fully to understand about muscle testing and what goes on in a kinesiology session, it is necessary first to understand something about subtle energy and the other concepts in this section. All kinesiology systems work with meridians and elements, but not all systems make use of some of the other concepts that are described.

Energy

Many kinesiologists talk about 'energy'. Sometimes they mean the usual definition of this – action, force, vigour, but more commonly it is short for subtle energy. The Concise Oxford Dictionary defines subtle as: 'tenuous or rarefied.... evasive, mysterious, hard to grasp or trace... making fine distinctions'. Subtle energy is a loose term used to describe any energy that is not specifically recognized and categorized by conventional scientific knowledge.

In her book *Energy Medicine* Donna Eden describes this energy as:

> ... the common medium of the body, mind and soul. Its wavelengths, rates of vibration, and patterns of pulsation form their shared vocabulary.

Just as the body has a physical system, it is understood by Chinese Medicine and Ayurvedic practitioners to have a subtle energy system, not recognised in general by science and medicine. The subtle energy system interacts with the physical body, but its essence is vibrational rather than physical. Other subtle energy concepts include subtle bodies, chakras, nadis and, most importantly for an understanding of kinesiology, meridians.

Some kinesiologies (such as Integrated Healing) work explicitly and extensively with the subtle energy system, whereas others (for example Applied Kinesiology) focus on working with meridians.

Subtle Bodies

Almost everyone recognises that human beings are not just physical bodies, but many traditions and therapies have a complex theory of subtle bodies to explain this additional 'something'. There is some disagreement about how many subtle bodies there are and what they are called. Most writers on this subject accept that, as well as there being a physical body, there is also an etheric body, an astral or emotional body, one or more mental bodies and a spiritual body. Many systems include additional bodies. Because of the inter-relation between the bodies, when one of them is disturbed, it affects the other bodies and can lead to physical problems and psychological distress.

Chakras

In Sanskrit chakra means 'disk' or 'wheel', which is how the chakras often appear to clairvoyants. Chakras are viewed as subtle energy centres linking different parts of the subtle energy system together. Some kinesiologies make little use of the concept of chakras, whereas others (such as Optimum Health Balance) make extensive use of them.

Most writers in this field believe that there are seven major chakras: the base chakra, the abdominal chakra, the solar plexus chakra, the heart chakra, the throat chakra, the brow or third eye chakra and the crown chakra. There are also many minor chakras, known as nadis. Each chakra is seen as having particular characteristics (such as emotional qualities, colour, sound, and so on) associated with it. Each chakra is also linked to a particular organ of the endocrine system. So, for instance, the throat chakra is related to the thyroid gland (located in the throat) and is associated with the emotions of shyness and paranoia. The brow chakra is associated with the pituitary gland (the master gland of the hormonal system) and with the emotions of anger and rage. Chakras also have other qualities, so, for example, the brow chakra is also associated with intuition.

Acupuncture Meridians

The meridian system is a central concept for most kinesiology systems. Meridians were first identified by Chinese practitioners thousands of years ago. They are seen as forming a subtle energy grid that supports and integrates the different aspects of each individual: physical, emotional, mental and spiritual. The meridian energy system distributes Chi energy or life force to the body and this energy carries with it (or possibly even is) information to allow all the parts to function harmoniously. Imbalances in this system can lead to acute or chronic ill health, as the life force energy is not fed correctly to the tissues and cells of the physical body.

In classical oriental medicine there are fourteen major meridian lines. There are two meridian lines on the midline of the body: the governing vessel running up the back of the torso, and the central or conception vessel running up the front of the torso. The other twelve meridians all run bilaterally on the surface of the body. These meridians are named after specific organs (e.g. the liver meridian, the small intestine meridian), but are not necessarily on or near the named organ. For example, the lung meridian runs down the inner arm to the thumb, one meridian on each arm.

The 14 meridians are:

- Central Meridian
- Governing Meridian
- Stomach Meridian
- Spleen Meridian
- Heart Meridian
- Small Intestine Meridian
- Bladder Meridian
- Kidney Meridian
- Circulation-Sex Meridian
- Triple Warmer Meridian
- Gall Bladder Meridian
- Liver Meridian
- Lung Meridian
- Large Intestine Meridian

The acupuncture meridians may relate directly to the health of the internal organ associated with it, although it is possible for the meridian to be out of balance and yet the related organ to be healthy. However if a meridian is continually out of balance it is likely that the organ itself will eventually be affected.

There are various points along each of the acupuncture meridians, and skilled practitioners can 'feel' the location of these points. These points have also been mapped electronically. They are the points that are needled in an acupuncture session. The points are numbered starting with number 1. So, the central meridian runs up the midline of the torso from point 1 (known as central Vessel 1 or Cv 1) at the perineum to Cv 24 just below the lower lip on the midline.

The number of points on each meridian can vary, although where the meridians are bilateral, the meridians are mirror images of each other. So, in the case of the lung meridian, point 1 (Lung1 or Lu1) is on the upper front of the chest close to the top of the arm and Lu 11 is on the thumb. The left side meridian starts with Lu1 on the left side and ends with Lu 11 on the left thumb; the right-sided meridian starts with Lu1 on the right side and ends with Lu 11 on the right thumb.

Acupuncturists insert fine needles into these points, whereas kinesiologists use other methods, including touching or tapping. Whatever technique is used, the aim is the same: to balance the flow of energy within the meridians.

For a long time the power of acupuncture was dismissed by Western medicine, because acupuncture theory did not fit with the medical understanding of how the body functions. However, gradually some doctors began to find that acupuncture could work for pain relief. As the body of evidence for the success of acupuncture with adults, babies and animals mounted, medical researchers began to consider the possibility of these subtle energy concepts more carefully, although many feel acupuncture works through the nervous system in some way. In fact, the reality of meridians and acupuncture points is becoming more evident in the availability of electrical devices which are used to locate acupuncture points. The electrical resistance of acupuncture points seems to be lower than that of the surrounding skin area. This suggests a real physical presence for acupuncture points.

Meridians And Muscles

In kinesiology each meridian is associated with one or more muscles. For example, the central meridian is associated with the supraspinatus. The spleen meridian is associated with five muscles: latissimus dorsi, lower trapezius, middle trapezius, opponens pollicis longus and triceps. Each of the basic fourteen muscles used in kinesiology (see page 17 is related to a meridian, so in testing the muscle you are also accessing information about that meridian:

Basic Fourteen Muscles	Meridian
Supraspinatus	Central
Teres major	Governing
Pectoralis major calvicular	Stomach
Latissimus dorsi	Spleen
Subscapularis	Heart
Quadriceps	Small Intestine

Peroneus	Bladder
Psoas	Kidney
Gluteus medius	Circulation-Sex
Teres minor	Triple Warmer
Anterior deltoid	Gall Bladder
Pectoralis major sternal	Liver
Anterior serratus	Lung
Fascia lata	Large intestine

Acupuncturists feel pulses to establish which meridians are out of balance, whereas kinesiologists use muscle testing, working with the meridian-muscle connection to establish which meridians need attention. So, for example, if the psoas muscle unlocks when muscle tested, it means (among other things) that there is likely to be an imbalance in the kidney meridian.

Elements

In traditional Chinese Medicine the material world is seen to be made up of five elements:

- Wood
- Fire
- Earth
- Metal
- Water

The five elements interact and have specific relationships with each other. Each element also has a relationship with a season, a stage in the life cycle of humans and animals. Particular elements are more prominent at particular times of the year and at particular times of our lives. Each element also has specific emotions, sounds, colours, taste, parts of the body, etc. associated with it. There are particular questions associated with each element. An individual can have too much or too little of an element within their life and their body. An imbalance in a particular element is likely to result in specific types of illnesses.

The wood element is associated with spring, with birth and the early years of life. It is also associated with the colour green and with rancidity, sourness and anger. A wood-type question is: Do you have enough roots to sustain your growth; and enough fuel to sustain your passions? People suffering from repeated imbalances in the wood element are likely to suffer from headaches, conjunctivitis and anxiety.

By contrast the fire element is associated with summer, the colour red, bitterness (both as a taste and an emotion) and joy. Once again it is possible to have too much or too little of this element in your life. Fire questions include: Are you too cold, unable to be passionate? Fire element imbalances can lead to insomnia, hearing problems and a lack of joy in life.

Earth is the element associated with late summer, the colour yellow, dampness, humidity, sweetness and the emotions of sympathy and empathy. People who have too little of the earth element in their life are selfish and focussed solely on what they want. People who have too much are constantly at the beck and call of others, putting others needs before their own in an unhealthy way.

The metal element is associated with grief, white, autumn, dryness and pungency. Questions associated with this element include: Are you too hard on yourself? and What have you lost? It is also associated with rationality, precision, self-control and a tendency to pessimism.

The water element is associated with decline and the end of life. It is also associated with the winter months. This element is associated with fear. It is important to have a certain amount of fear in life, otherwise we would put ourselves into unnecessary danger, but too much fear and anxiety can be stifling. The colour blue is associated with the water element, so wearing more blue may bring this element back into balance. However, if there is too much energy in water, reducing the amount of blue worn is likely to be beneficial. A cool climate is associated with this element too.

Each element is said to be the mother of (or the creator of) the one that follows. So, wood creates fire, which creates earth which creates metal which creates water which creates wood. The cycle continues and continues with no element being any more important than any other element. This is known as the creation cycle.

There is another important cycle known as the control cycle:

- Wood controls earth
- Earth controls water
- Water controls fire
- Fire controls metal
- Metal controls wood

These two cycles are used by many kinesiologists in the work they do to help rebalance the energy system.

Yin And Yang

Yin and yang are fundamental concepts in the oriental view of the world. Everything manifests through an interplay of opposites: yin and yang. Everything has yin and yang qualities within them, but the balance between yin and yang varies. Yang qualities include expansiveness, dryness, masculinity, lightness, heat and hollowness. Yin qualities include femininity, receptivity, darkness, coolness and solidity. Each meridian is seen to be predominantly yin or predominantly yang. Each yang meridian needs its paired yin meridian for its completion. Each yin meridian needs to be balanced by its paired yang meridian.

Each meridian flows in a particular direction. In general yin meridians flow from the feet towards the head, and yang meridians flow from the head to the feet.

Each pair is also linked to an element, except for the fire element which has four meridians associated with it:

Element	Yang Meridian	Yin Meridian
Wood	Gall Bladder	Liver
Fire	Small Intestine	Heart
	Triple Water	Circulation-Sex
Earth	Stomach	Spleen
Metal	Large Intestine	Lung
Water	Bladder	Kidney

Some kinesiology systems focus on the traditional five elements, but others, such as Applied Physiology and Health Kinesiology also include the central and governing meridians and treat these as a separate element.

Eight Extra Meridians

Some kinesiologists also work with eight extra meridians. These are believed to be the first meridians that develop in the foetus and carry the baby's genetic inheritance. They run deep within the body and provide the other meridians with life force energy. Wayne Topping (see page 173 has developed muscle tests involving these eight extra meridians, which allow the five element meridians to be balanced at the same time using emotions, nutrients, biokinetic exercises (see page 43), etc.

Aura/Auric Field

Aura, or auric field, refers to a field of subtle, luminous radiation surrounding a person. Some people believe they can see this. Some kinesiologists will test for the strength of the person's aura and may scan the aura looking for holes in the energy field that need repairing, although other kinesiology systems do not consider the aura at all.

Energetic Cords/Karmic Strings

This is another concept that is not part of some kinesiology systems. Where it is used, the understanding is that there are connections between people that directly affect a person's health and well-being. One person may try consciously or subconsciously to bind someone else to them and dictate the course of the other person's life. These terms recognise that this can operate at an unseen, energetic level as well as more obviously through verbal communication and behaviour. These energetic connections can come about as a result of an argument not satisfactorily being resolved or a parent not allowing a child to become independent or, some practitioners would argue, from a past life encounter.

Muscle Testing

George Goodheart (see page 03) started by testing the functional integrity of a particular muscle or muscles involved with the shoulder, but kinesiology testing has evolved to use the muscle testing as an indicator of energy changes within the body. For this reason it is sometimes called muscle monitoring, and practitioners will refer to an indicator muscle (see page 18) or a clear circuit muscle indicator (Three in One).

Many practitioners also prefer the term muscle monitoring because testing implies something that the client can pass or fail, and clients can easily jump to the conclusion that a weak muscle response is a failure, rather than simply an indication of a particular state. Some practitioners also talk about muscle feedback for the same reason.

Testing A Muscle

Whether practitioners call it muscle testing, muscle monitoring or muscle feedback, the basic process is the same. Muscle testing is a painless procedure involving the practitioner applying gentle pressure to specific parts of the body (often arms and legs) to test the response of the underlying muscle. Many of the muscles can be tested standing, sitting or lying down. All muscles can be tested while the client wears a reasonable amount of clothing.

The particular part of the body involved is placed in a specific position, in order, as far as possible, to isolate the muscle that is being tested. The body normally uses several different muscles to perform any movement, so testing an individual muscle is not in practice usually possible, but kinesiologists work to isolate a muscle as best they can. The tested muscle will either easily be able to resist the pressure from the practitioner or will give way. Sometimes the muscle will not give way, but not hold either; it will be spongy. This is often because the client is trying to recruit other muscles. For example, when a weak leg muscle is being tested, the subject sometimes automatically tips their hips to engage other muscles and compensate for the weakness.

The kinesiologist uses this on/off response to gain information about what is happening and what is needed to restore balance. Because of the inter-relationship between muscles, meridians and body systems (see page 10, this information applies not only to the muscle being tested but more frequently is used to give valuable information about other imbalances within the body and the necessary procedures to correct them.

The pressure applied by the practitioner starts gently and gradually increases. If the practitioner suddenly applies the full pressure, the muscle is likely to give way and produce an inaccurate test. The Touch for Health manual advises using no more than 2 lbs of pressure, for no more than 2 seconds. Applying pressure for longer than this can fatigue the muscle so that it gives way. In practice, the amount of pressure used varies from practitioner to practitioner. Some kinesiologists use very light pressure, whereas others prefer firmer pressure.

Sometimes the muscle will give way a little before responding. Some clients need to feel the pressure of the test before they respond. This is a reason for applying the pressure slowly as this gives the muscle chance to react. The Touch for Health manual specifies that the muscle needs to lock within 2 inches of the starting position. If it locks after more movement, this suggests that other muscles are being recruited.

The kinesiologist will usually ask the client to 'hold' just before testing. At one time practitioners often used the word 'resist' rather than 'hold', but it became clear that the word 'resist' encouraged people to believe that if the muscle did not lock, they had failed in some way. Strong men are often astounded when their muscle weakens under the gentle testing pressure, but this is because the test is not a test for the strength of the muscle but is an indicator of some imbalance within the body.

Some kinesiologists (e.g. Three in One facilitators) will test both arms (or legs) simultaneously. They do so "to be sure there is agreement between the right and left hemispheres" (*Tools of the Trade Book 1*).

Some kinesiologists also test the muscle both in extension and in contraction. Each muscle has a range of movement; testing in both these ways means that it is tested at both ends of the range. So, for example, the anterior deltoid (a front shoulder muscle) is tested when the arm is at about 30 degrees to the body and also when the arm is by the side of the body. This is seen as a way of accessing information from both hemispheres of the brain.

Binary Testing

Originally the terms 'strong' and 'weak' were used to describe whether or not a muscle held during testing. This is probably as a result of kinesiology's origins in chiropractic, where muscle testing was undertaken to establish the physical integrity of muscles.

As many kinesiologists are using the muscle test as an indicator (of the state of a meridian, stress, energy imbalances, etc.) using the term 'weak' is inappropriate: the muscle response is what it is, giving information about what is going on for the person and helping the practitioner establish what needs to be done for the client.

Other terms are now more generally used to avoid this negative connotation, such as:

- Locked/unlocked
- On/off
- Facilitated/inhibited
- Muscle change
- Yes/no

Because there are two possible results to the muscle test (on/off), this is sometimes referred to as binary muscle testing.

Analogue & Holographic Testing

In recent years some kinesiology systems have started using analogue and/or holographic testing rather than binary testing.

Analogue testing was developed by Alan Sales (see page 79). He noticed that when he tested a muscle through the range of its motion (from contraction to extension), there would sometimes be a 'blip' in the smooth change of position of the arm or leg being tested. Alan saw this as representing how locked or unlocked a muscle was. So instead of having 0 (unlocked) and 100 (locked) for a muscle test, he could now get a percentage. This allowed for a more nuanced approach and was a way of finding imbalances that the binary system might not reveal. It would be unwieldy to have to test every muscle in this way, so Alan identified a finger mode (see page 21) that could be used instead. When this mode is in circuit, the muscle will unlock if the circuit is anything from 1% to 100% out of balance. Alan used the analogy of digital and analogue format in audio. When you listen to a piece of music in digital, all the sounds outside the set bandwidth are deleted. It is either there or not there. In analogue, you hear the sound at the bandwidth and also the sounds close by.

Richard Utt (see page 63) developed holographic testing. Each muscle has a strong, primary relationship with a specific meridian, and this is tested in the binary mode, but the muscle also has a secondary connection with all the other meridians, and these are tested through the whole range of its motion. There are seven positions in which the muscle can be tested, and the muscle can be tested going towards contraction or extension, so this gives tests relating to each of the fourteen meridians (see page 09) used in kinesiology and in traditional Chinese Five Element Theory.

42 Muscles

Muscle testing in kinesiology has evolved so that now 42 different muscles may be tested. Kinesiology text books and manuals offer detailed information on the placement of the body so that, as far as possible, an individual muscle is tested. The 42 muscles are:

- Supraspinatus
- Teres major
- Pectoralis major clavicular
- Levator scapulae
- Anterior flexors (neck)
- Posterior flexors (neck)
- Brachioradialis
- Latissimus dorsi
- Lower trapezius
- Middle trapezius
- Opponens pollicis longus
- Triceps
- Subscapularis
- Quadriceps
- Abdominals
- Peroneus
- Sacrospinalis
- Tibials (anterior and posterior)
- Posterior tibial
- Psoas
- Upper trapezius

- Iliacus
- Gluteus medius
- Adductors
- Piriformis
- Gluteus maximus
- Teres minor
- Sartorius
- Gracilis
- Soleus
- Gastrocnemius
- Anterior deltoid
- Popliteus
- Pectoralis major sterna
- Rhomboids
- Anterior serratus
- Coracobrachialis
- Deltoids
- Diaphragm
- Fascia lata
- Hamstrings
- Quadratus lamborum

Some kinesiology systems use additional muscles, notably Professional Kinesiology Provider. PKP has added additional muscles and includes over 100 potential muscle tests.

Basic 14 Muscles

Although there are 42 standard muscles that can be tested, 14 of these are used much more commonly. These are:

- Supraspinatus
- Teres major
- Pectoralis major clavicular
- Latissimus dorsi
- Subscapularis
- Quadriceps
- Peroneus
- Psoas
- Gluteus medius
- Teres minor
- Anterior deltoid
- Pectoralis major sternal
- Anterior serratus
- Fascia lata

Each of these 14 muscles relates to one of the meridians (see page 09) and so can be used to test specifically for that meridian.

17

Indicator Muscles

Some practitioners always start with a 14 muscle balance, testing one muscle per meridian, but some practitioners only use one or two muscles in a session. This is because the muscle is being used as an indicator muscle. It is not being solely tested to establish its physical integrity or even the state of its related meridian but is being used to gain a range of other information about the whole system, such as supplement needs, chakra imbalances, neurotransmitter problems, psychological issues, past traumatic events, etc. etc.

Because indicator muscles are repeatedly tested during a session, some muscles are more appropriate than others. Three In One recommends the anterior deltoid (front shoulder muscle) or the pectoralis major clavicular (upper chest muscle), whereas Health Kinesiology practitioners tend to use the brachioradialis (lower arm muscle). Whatever muscle or muscle is chosen, it needs to be a naturally strong muscle that is easy for the client to hold in position and that is not injured in any way.

Normally, before the real work begins, pre-checks are run (see page 25) to make sure that this indicator muscle is functioning properly.

Some kinesiologies that use verbal questioning (page 22) use the indicator muscle to show an answer to a yes/no question - a locked response means 'yes' and an unlocked or weak response means 'no'. So, for example if the query was whether the client would benefit from taking a vitamin C supplement a kinesiologist who uses verbal questioning would ask a question and test the muscle. The question could be phrased in various ways, but could be, for example: Would it be beneficial to take a vitamin C supplement? A locked response indicates that the person should take the supplement (yes), an unlocked response indicates that the client would not benefit from this supplement (no).

Other kinesiologists are looking for a change in the indicator muscle: a strong muscle, now testing weak or a weak muscle, now testing strong. A kinesiologist who is checking for an indicator change will usually start with a weak muscle response and then check the vitamin C (the client has the supplement in the mouth, on the body or in the hand) to see if it will give a strong muscle on testing. A strong response once again means that the client would benefit from taking it.

Surrogate Testing

Small babies, the mentally and physically handicapped, frail old people and animals can all be tested using surrogate testing. The practitioner will muscle test someone (the surrogate) who is holding or touching the client. It is commonly thought to work best if the surrogate and the subject (baby, animal, handicapped person, etc.) have a relationship, e.g. a mother being a surrogate for her child, but it can also work where there is no pre-existing relationship.

Once I was giving a talk on kinesiology and the question of testing babies came up. I was talking about allergies at the time, so I tested one lady who showed she was reacting to chocolate. Then I tested someone else who was not. Next I got them to hold hands and used the second lady as a surrogate. Now muscle testing her showed up the chocolate reaction of her friend. This produced a lot of interest and eventually we had twenty people holding hands with the lady with the chocolate reaction at one end. I tested the person at the other end, who did not have a chocolate allergy herself, and once again the chocolate problem showed through. This was really a party trick, as you only need one person to act as a surrogate to test another person or animal, but nevertheless it clearly and dramatically demonstrates the phenomenon of surrogate testing.

Self-Testing

Sometimes, rather than testing the client's muscles, practitioners will use themselves as a surrogate, testing a muscle of their own, usually a finger. This can be much faster than testing the client's muscles. It is also used if, for some reason, the client cannot be tested directly and there is not a suitable surrogate available. Practitioners also use self-testing to work on themselves when another practitioner is not available.

Intention And Clarity

The importance of clarity and intention is evident in surrogate testing and when practitioners use self-testing to establish information about clients. The kinesiologist has to be clear that in these situations only information relevant to the subject will be accessed.

Under Energy And Over Energy

A meridian (see page 09) can be unbalanced because of over or under energy. Alarm points (see below) and the pulse check (see below) are ways of establishing whether or not there is over energy or under energy in the meridian. This can also be established by verbal questioning (see page 22). Although many kinesiology systems have a preference for working with under energy, some (e.g. Health Kinesiology) have a preference for focussing on the meridians with over energy. In Touch for Health one or more of the meridians will be re-balanced. In many kinesiology systems the imbalance will be added to circuit (see page 20), rather than being dealt with in isolation.

Alarm Points

Alarm points are a test of over energy (see above). Each meridian has associated alarm points on the torso – some are on the midline and some are bilateral. The points are not necessarily located on the meridian itself. A previously strong indicator muscle is tested while the alarm points are held. If the muscle unlocks, this means there is over energy in the meridian associated with that alarm point or points.

The Pulse Check

An alternative way to establish which meridian (if any) has over energy in it is to use the pulse check. The pulse area of the wrist relates to 12 meridians (not central and governing). There are 3 pulse spots on each wrist which can be held lightly or deeply:

- Left wrist - light touch relates to small intestine, gall bladder and bladder meridians.
- Left wrist - deep touch relates to hear, liver and kidney meridians.
- Right wrist - light touch relates to large intestine, stomach and triple warmer meridians.
- Right wrist - deep touch relates to lung, spleen and circulation-sex meridians.

An experienced practitioner particularly one who is trained in Chinese medicine can obtain a lot of information from feeling the pulses. Kinesiologist ask clients to hold each pulse spot in turn (either lightly or firmly) while they test a leg muscle. If the muscle switches off or is spongy, this indicates over energy in the related meridian.

This over energy can be corrected by using acupressure points to sedate the meridian.

Polarity And Testing

Some kinesiologists use two fingers when testing and/or correcting, because they see the fingers as having a negative or positive polarity. By using two adjacent fingers the effect of this polarity is cancelled out.

Pause Lock / Stacking / Adding To Circuit / Circuit Retaining Mode

There are many different terms used, but they all are variations of pause lock. The originator of pause lock was the late Dr Alan Beardall. Pause lock is used by many different kinesiology systems. Its use can make the session much less painful or stressful for the client. For example, the client may have a pain in their wrist that they only experience when they hold it in a certain position. If the practitioner does not use verbal questioning (see page 22) nor pause lock, the client would have to stay in the painful position while the issues and corrections involved with the pain are established. Similarly to address a phobia, the client would have to think about the phobic situation continuously; a highly stressful thing to do. In addition, if the client's mind wandered from the stressful thought, testing would become inaccurate, but the practitioner would not necessarily be able to tell that the client was no longer thinking about the stressful situation. Using pause lock means that there is still a snapshot of the thought even if the client's mind wanders.

In pause lock the energetic information is locked or stacked into a 'virtual databank'. The original way to do pause lock was using the legs. In the painful wrist example, the client would bend their arm to stimulate the pain, while the legs would be kept straight and be put together and then put apart by the practitioner. Then the wrist could be put in a more comfortable position, but as long as the legs stayed apart, all the testing would relate to the wrist pain. Once the legs are brought back together again and left there, that information or energetic pattern is lost.

Since the original development other ways of achieving pause lock have been established. The practitioner may, for example, use the fingers, jaws or the roof of the mouth. Often practitioners will use their own bodies rather than that of clients, as this removes the need to give the client detailed instructions about how to do it.

Pause lock is also used to stack or add information to an issue or problem. Stacking recognizes that often there may be several different causes or triggers for a problem. The practitioner may want to register all these different triggers and look for the one thing that is needed to correct them.

For example, if the client was shy and wanted to increase their self-confidence, he (or she) would think about a situation which triggered the shyness. This would be locked in with pause lock. Now the client does not have to keep thinking about the stressful situation. The practitioner might then use finger modes (see page 21) to establish that something is needed from the emotional realm. Testing might show the statement *I hate my mother* is relevant to this. This statement would be added to circuit - while the client said the statement, he (or the practitioner) would close and immediately open his legs again (or use one of the other pause lock techniques using the fingers, roof of the mouth, etc.) Once again the practitioner would use the finger modes to establish what else is needed – at this stage the testing relates both to the shyness and to the mother hatred. Now, for example, a biochemical problem might be indicated, say, a calcium deficiency. Again this would be added to the databank using pause lock. This process would carry on until no further finger modes showed. Eventually muscle testing will show that there is nothing further to add (either using the finger mode for 'more' or through verbal questioning). Then the correction is carried out for the last thing that has been found and that, like pushing a domino, corrects all the other issues (events, emotions, imbalances, etc.) that have been stacked.

Once this has been done, the pause lock is removed - in this case the legs are closed. Now the original problem is retested - the client thinks about a situation which makes him shy and an indicator muscle is tested. If the work has been effective, the muscle will test strong, and the client will say that thinking about the situation is much less stressful.

Sometimes this process needs to be repeated again for other aspects of the original issue. For example, the treatment so far might have helped the client to be less shy in a work situation, but not in a social situation. The process can be carried out again (either in the same session or in a subsequent session) to deal with the social shyness triggers.

Biocomputer

Many kinesiologists refer to muscle testing as having a dialogue with the body's 'biocomputer' and upgrading programming or reprogramming the biocomputer. This concept was originally developed by Dr Alan Beardall, a US chiropractor and kinesiologist. They may also talk about files, directories, sub-directories and computer readouts.

Finger Modes

Finger modes were also developed by Dr Alan Beardall. He discovered these because he was looking for a simple way to identify which is the optimum treatment for a particular person at a particular time. Finger modes are specific combinations of finger positions, which relate to specific body systems, correction procedures, and so on. His original discovery came about because he had identified a weak muscle in a patient. He stopped to record this result and then retested the muscle. The muscle tested strong. He was surprised at this but noticed that the patient had several fingers touching each other. He retested the muscle with the fingers not touching, and once again the muscle tested weak. Because of the way the finger modes were discovered, most kinesiologists believe that in some way they are hard wired into the body rather than just being a matter of convention or intention. Dr Beardall was sadly killed in a car accident in England in 1987.

There are many different finger modes each involving placing one or more fingers against other parts of the hand. For example, the tip of the middle finger placed against the tip of the thumb indicates nutritional or biochemical problems. The finger mode is usually carried out by the kinesiologist, mainly because this is quicker than explaining to the client exactly how to place the fingers. While the finger mode is held, a muscle is tested. If there is a change, this means that (in this case) the problem needs nutritional or biochemical corrections/input. If the tip of the index finger had been placed against the tip of the thumb, this would indicate a structural problem when there was a change in the muscle. If there is no change, this indicates

21

that this particular area is not relevant at this time. Sometimes two finger modes might show as being relevant, in which case the practitioner would probably use the priority finger mode (see page 21 and 32) to establish the energy system's preference.

Finger modes can be used in many different ways, for example, to determine priority (see page 32), establish whether more work is needed at the current time, to decide which type of correction is needed for a particular goal, etc.

Not all kinesiologies use finger modes to the same extent. Professional Kinesiology Provider makes extensive use of finger modes, whereas Health Kinesiology relies on verbal questioning (see below) to access the same level of information. Some kinesiologists use a mixture of finger modes and verbal questioning.

Formatting

Richard Utt (see Applied Physiology) initially developed the concept of accessing specific brain structures and functions by using a combination of acupoints and mudras (hand or finger modes) from yoga, a system he called acupressure formatting. It is now used extensively in other kinesiologies too. For example, NeuroEnergetic Kinesiology and AcuNeuroSync/LEAP make extensive use of formatting.

Practitioners use a combination of acupuncture points (see page 09) and finger modes (see page 21) to pinpoint a particular organ, biochemical pathway, neurotransmitter, emotional component, etc. So for example, if practitioners want to check the energetic functioning of the amygdala (see page 32), they would use a combination of two finger modes (one for anatomy, one for physiology) and a precise acupuncture point for the amygdala. If this same acupuncture point is touched in conjunction with a different finger mode or finger modes, it will be testing something different.

This combination of finger mode(s) and acupuncture points is referred to as a format. While the format is in place, an indicator muscle is tested. A change in muscle response indicates that there is an imbalance that needs addressing. This would then usually be added into circuit (see page 20).

Verbal Questioning

Some kinesiology systems, such as health kinesiology, make extensive use of verbal muscle testing. The response of a correctly positioned muscle to light pressure can be either to lock or unlock. The kinesiologist uses this to ask verbal questions: the locked response of the muscle indicates "yes" and the unlocked or spongy response indicates "no". The practitioner will then use systematic questioning with the muscle testing to establish what technique or techniques are needed from the many possible procedures that the practitioner learnt during training. The practitioner can also use verbal questioning in conjunction with muscle testing to establish an exercise or a diet and supplement programme for the client. Because of the ability to access information through muscle testing, this programme will be tailored specifically for the individual concerned. Some kinesiologists prefer to use statements rather than questions, so might say "That is correct" rather than "Is that correct?"

Some kinesiologists do not use verbal questioning at all or only in a limited way. Instead they rely on accessing information by testing a muscle whilst touching specific points on the body or using a finger mode and/or formatting.

Overview Of The Session

People consult a kinesiologist for a variety of reasons. These include physical symptoms and illnesses. Sometimes people seek help because doctors are unable to make a diagnosis or are dismissive; drugs may not be working well or have unacceptable side effects. Some people want to avoid drugs altogether. Some people seek help because they feel stressed, lack confidence and do not feel in control of their life or are unhappy with the way it is going. Sometimes people seek help with particular skills, such as reading, spelling, dance, sport, etc.

Kinesiology can work to help people reach their potential whatever that may be. I once had a child with cerebral palsy brought to see me. He was 6 years old and had very limited speech. His mother recognised that he would always have cerebral palsy but wanted him to speak better. She believed this would be good for him and good for their relationship if his speech improved. Within a couple of sessions his speech and ability to communicate had improved dramatically, although it was still less than that of a normal six year old child. Through the phenomenon of surrogate testing (see page 18), babies, frail old people, the physically and mentally handicapped, and animals can all be helped.

There are, however, huge variations in the way kinesiologists practice. Some are happy to focus on symptoms and medical conditions, whereas others prefer to focus on balancing the body's energy system, trusting that this will bring about healing. Some practitioners see themselves as educators rather than therapists. Some practitioners work extensively with past lives and divine purpose, while others do not include these concepts in their work. The section on the different kinesiology systems (see page 46 onwards) looks at this in more detail.

Meridian Energy System Balance

The concept of balance is central to all kinesiology systems. Kinesiologists believe that ill health is caused by imbalances within the energy system, especially the meridian energy system.

Balance is not a fixed, static state. It involves an uninterrupted flow of yin and yang energies (see page 12) through the meridians, producing an optimum level of each at any given time, though one will always be dominant.

At different hours of the day different meridians will be prominent (see page160). Different situations in the external world affect how the system is at any point: what is right now is unlikely to be the best at 2 am in the morning, or when you are competing in a marathon. Ideally the meridian energy system is in dynamic balance, changing and rebalancing according to internal and external circumstances. However, for many people the meridian energy is more often out of balance than in balance, leading to health problems. Many things can lead to imbalances in the meridian energy, including psychological stress, pollution, inadequate nutrition, etc. Kinesiologists work to redress these imbalances, so promoting good health and well-being. In an ideal state the energy system would constantly be adjusting and readjusting according to internal and external circumstances so that it is always moving towards balance.

Sadly many people do not experience how good this feels as their energy systems are habitually in an unbalanced state. One of the great promises of kinesiology is to help the whole person achieve the habit of dynamic balance. This results in good health and emotional well-being. In the Touch for Health Manual John Thie wrote:

> We are not seeking a static, "ultimate" state of health ... We are seeking to help people live more fully in the moment, appreciating the dynamic dance of life and the flow of energy and creativity. (page xix)

Kinesiology practitioners work to re-establish balance and there are many different protocols, procedures and techniques aimed at achieving this.

Each time the energy system is balanced it puts it in a better position to deal with changes and challenges in the future, but there is always more work to do. I sometimes used to joke with clients that, when there was no longer any work to do, they would disappear in a puff of smoke!

The Start Of A Kinesiology Session

When a person sees a kinesiologist, the kinesiologist may refer to it as a session or a treatment or a balance.

The first thing most practitioners do is to take a detailed case history and explain about kinesiology and what to expect from the session, although if you are having a Touch for Health session with a friend this may not happen.

There is no standard kinesiology format - different kinesiology systems teach different approaches, and then individual practitioners may well vary what they do within that. Some practitioners will focus on symptoms (asking about problems), some will ask clients about their goals and what they want to achieve from the kinesiology sessions, and some will ask about both.

In general clients do not need to take off their clothes, although sometimes the practitioner might ask the client to remove bulky items of clothing so that a particular acupuncture point can be located accurately. Practitioners often use a treatment couch (also known as a table), and clients lie on this while the session is carried out. If a client is unable to lie down, the session can usually be adapted so that the client can be treated standing or sitting down and in fact, some practitioners prefer this anyway.

Pre-Checks

Most kinesiology systems use some initial testing procedure, often known as pre-checks. The point of the pre-checks is to establish that the practitioner has a reliable muscle in the clear. This means that the muscle when tested will respond appropriately; it will not lock (see page 15) all the time or be spongy all the time; it will not stay locked when it should unlock or vice versa.

Many kinesiologists will run some tests that challenge different aspects of the person and their energy system. For example, an emotional challenge might be to ask the person to think about something upsetting. When an indicator muscle is tested in this situation, the muscle should unlock.

A verbal test challenge might be to ask the person to say 'yes' and then 'no'. The normal response is for the muscle to hold/lock for 'yes' and unlock for 'no'.

The physical challenge is often to turn the muscle off by pinching the belly of a muscle. If the same muscle is tested immediately afterwards, the correct response is for the muscle to unlock.

Placing a magnet on a muscle and testing it, should result in either a locked or unlocked response depending on which pole of the magnet is against the skin. This provides a test of the electro-magnetic system of the body.

The indicator muscle needs to respond appropriately to these pre-tests, so that the practitioner can have confidence that when the test is for something with an unknown answer (e.g. is there over energy in the lung meridian?) the muscle will give an accurate response - tell it as it is.

If the pre-checks do not give the correct results, various remedial actions will need to be carried out. These can include drinking water, having specific spots on the body touched or rubbed, etc.

In Touch for Health the following are done before these pre-checks:

- Central meridian zip ups
- Switching
- Tune in

In Health Kinesiology the thymus area (over the breast bone and below the collar bone) may be tapped before carrying out the pre-checks.

These procedures are designed to make it more likely that the energy system will be balanced and that the pre-checks will give the correct results.

Permission To Proceed

Once the initial balancing procedure is complete many kinesiologists will ask permission to proceed either generally or for a specific issue. So, for example, Three In One Concept facilitators usually ask:

> "Do we have permission to test this issue?"
> And
> "Is there any reason NOT to work with this person?"

Health kinesiology practitioners usually ask:

> "Do we have energy permission to work together now?"
> And
> "Is there any reason why not?"

Although the practitioners come from different kinesiology systems and so frame the question slightly differently, they are essentially asking the same question.

Deciding What To Do

When I was working as a kinesiologist I often felt that the other person's inner wisdom/energy system would check me out, as we started to work, to assess what skills and expertise I had. Once this checking out was completed, the analysis and work could be mapped out using the best I could offer for that client. Terry Larder (see page 67) describes it like this:

> An office can have a number of computers that are networked together and share information using the same software programmes. When the practitioner is in contact with the client, they become a network and the information and skills in the practitioner's virtual databank becomes available and understood by that of the client.

For this reason the session represents a partnership between the client and the practitioner, a pooling of joint history, knowledge, experiences and skills. This means that a client may experience very different sessions from different practitioners, even when both practitioners use the same kinesiology system.

Some practitioners will decide on the focus of the session through that initial discussion with the client. Other practitioners will encourage the client to decide on the problem or goal to be addressed. This usually follows detailed discussion with the practitioner in which the practitioner offers insights and suggestions, which may alter the client's perception and understanding, so that they will decide on a different problem or goal as the focus for the session.

Some practitioners will use muscle testing to decide on the appropriate goal for the session after a discussion with the client as to what they see as being important. This is particularly likely with practitioners who make extensive use of verbal questioning (such as Health Kinesiologists). Practitioners who take this approach believe that sometimes clients consciously or subconsciously avoid discussing important issues, because they feel fearful, embarrassed or guilty. Practitioners using muscle testing to establish the thrust of the work believe that muscle testing will only produce issues and goals that can safely be addressed, however much the client may be fearful initially.

Some practitioners will establish the goal through discussion and then use muscle testing to confirm this is the most appropriate focus for the session. This can be phrased in various ways, for example:

- Is this the best goal for the session?
- Is this the most appropriate thing to do right now?
- Is this the best goal in your highest good for now?

They then muscle test to find out whether the answer is 'yes' or 'no'.

Some practitioners also like to find the main emotion that goes with the goal using a five element chart (see page 11) or the Behavioural Barometer (see page 151).

Some practitioners will also test how ready the client is to change to achieve the goal. This question may be subdivided into asking, for example, about willingness on physical, emotional, mental and spiritual levels. If the commitment is not 100% on one or more of the levels, an Emotional Stress Release SR correction (see page 40) may be done. Another way of doing this is to ask through muscle testing if the client is ready to release the need for the problem, accept the benefits of change etc.

Some practitioners also ask the client to grade any problem or difficulty on a scale of 1 to 10, before the work begins. The grading can be used for many different types of symptoms, problems and goals, e.g. a relationship problem, back pain, difficulty reading, feeling confident, etc.

The client may also be asked to grade the problem at the end of the session, but this is not always appropriate. Often clients are not aware of any improvement immediately after the session. This could be because no change has happened, but often it is because the input from the session needs to be processed in some way before any improvement can be consciously experienced. It could also be that the client needs to be in the situation that normally triggers the problem in order to know if any change has happened.

Addressing The Problem/Goal

Once the goal or issue or symptoms have been decided, and the pre-checks have been completed, the rest of the work that is carried out is done in relation to the problem or goal that is being addressed. This means that there may be lots of different imbalances, but that muscle testing will only show up the ones related to the problem/goal.

What happens next varies considerably from kinesiology system to kinesiology system. Some systems make extensive use of finger modes (see page 21) and/or pause lock (see page 20), whereas others make much more use of verbal questioning (see page 22). There are many different correcting and rebalancing techniques depending on the training and expertise of the practitioner.

Client Insights

Frequently, as practitioners work bringing together the different strands that make up the session, clients will start to make connections for themselves; for example, they may realise why they have always behaved in a certain way around a particular person, or why they hate a particular colour. These points of recognition or understanding can be intense and satisfying for clients and enhance the healing process itself. That said, I personally have had clients who could not make sense of any of the sessions but still experienced great transformations in their lives. I am sure most other practitioners have had this experience too.

What Does It Mean?

Muscle testing is a skill that can be taught to anyone who wishes to learn and is prepared to put in an appropriate amount of effort and work, but the interpretation of the response depends on the type of kinesiology that is practiced.

It may seem strange that a muscle response in one system of kinesiology can mean something completely different in another kinesiology system. The best way to understand these apparent conflicts is to see the different kinesiology systems speaking different languages: the same word can mean different things in different languages, but all is well as long as it is clear which language is being spoken. Another way of looking at this is to view the practitioner as using a software programme that has been written to achieve a task. Each software programme is written differently and has different rules of use.

In the Touch for Health manual John Thie wrote:

> … what the test means and what we do about it has more to do with the context of the muscle-testing relationship between two people than it does with the precise observation of individual muscle response.
> Page 16

Finishing The Session

Most practitioners will check at the end of the session that it is appropriate to stop. There are various ways to do this, including using finger modes (page 21) or verbal questioning (page 22).

Depending on what has happened in the session, it may not be appropriate to stop work. For example, if the client has been working through some emotional issue, there may be some other aspect of it that needs addressing before the session is finished. If the session is likely to encourage physical healing, extra zinc or vitamin C may be needed; the client will need to know this and know what foods or supplements to take to support the healing process.

How Often Is Kinesiology Needed?

The frequency and number of sessions varies depending on how the practitioner works and what is being addressed. Many kinesiologists will use the muscle testing to establish when the client should return - sometimes this can be a week later, or treatments may even be several months apart. The number of sessions varies too and is not always related to the apparent gravity of the problem or symptoms.

Once the original issue that brought the client to the kinesiologist has been successfully addressed, many clients see the value of the work and decide to come back for regular maintenance appointments, seeking to address imbalances they may not even be aware of and so avoid more serious problems down the line.

Healing Crisis/ Healing Process

Sometimes people feel worse after a session. The most likely reason is that the body is processing information and energetic changes. Common responses include a flare up of existing physical symptoms, flu-like symptoms, spots, headaches, smelly sweat, vivid dreams and tiredness. If verbal questioning (see page 22) is being used, the practitioner can establish what can be expected. These symptoms will only last a few days at most. Integrated Healing has specific checks during a session to minimise the occurrence of healing crises.

There is usually a subtle difference between a healing crisis and an exacerbation of symptoms. The client may notice that their appetite is good and that they feel positive in spite of all the symptoms.

Does The Body Lie?

Some practitioners believe that the body never lies, and that muscle testing will always produce the correct response when carried out by a competent practitioner. This assumes the practitioner to be functioning at 100% all the time, but like any other job or activity, sometimes the practitioner will, for various reasons, not be 100% accurate and will make mistakes.

But, even if the practitioner is competent and is performing and reading the muscle testing response accurately, is the response itself always accurate?

Many practitioners believe that sometimes the body does lie and that part of the work that is undertaken is to remove the blocks and subterfuges that hinder accurate transmission of information through the muscle testing system. In this view, this may be because of fear or addiction, or because the energy system may have a different agenda from that of the practitioner and the client's conscious mind. Many kinesiology systems have specific techniques and procedures that work to overcome this.

Diagnosing Illnesses

Occasionally clients will ask therapists to diagnose a problem. They will say, for example: Do I have breast cancer? or Is my stomach ulcer caused by the helicobacter pylori bacteria?

Most kinesiologists are not qualified to make a medical diagnosis, and anyway the fundamental ideas of kinesiology lead the practitioner away from what is seen as a narrow approach to healing in the medical model. Kinesiologists prefer to look for imbalances in the energy system of the body.

The kinesiologist can help the client with stress around the idea of having a particular disease or dealing with the shock engendered by a medical diagnosis. This sort of work means that the client often can see more clearly what they need to do. At one time I was treating someone with severe epilepsy, who was having several fits a week in spite of her medication. Her fits stopped and she, of her own accord, decided to stop taking her medication. Subsequently she went for a routine hospital check-up. The consultant was horrified that she had stopped taking her medication and told her she must take it again She started the medication and within a week she was having fits again. Fortunately she phoned me for an appointment. This time the session focussed around the information that this powerful figure had given her that had become a self-fulfilling prophecy. Within a short time her fits had stopped again.

Most kinesiologists will also not test whether a client should stop a particular medication, and in most countries it is illegal for them to do so unless they have medical qualifications as well.

Some Important Concepts

The Triad Of Health

A central concept of many kinesiologies is the triad of health. This is envisaged as a triangle with three sides labelled structural, emotional (or mental) and biochemical (or just chemical). Each side is equally important and the three sides affect each other. For example, a structural problem such as an injured joint may have emotional/mental repercussions too. A problem in the biochemical area (such as an excess intake of a toxic mineral or an under production in the body of hydrochloric acid) can have structural and mental/emotional affects too. Any problem could have mental/emotional components and structural issues, all of which need to be addressed for complete healing to take place.

The triad of health does not have a place for spiritual considerations. Some kinesiologists see this as a weakness of the triad of health model, whereas others see spiritual issues as being outside the remit of the practitioner.

The Holographic Model

If you have a holographic image and cut it into pieces, each piece contains all the information from the original, so is capable of generating the full image. This contrasts with a normal image, where cutting it up destroys the full image. As you cut the holographic image into smaller and smaller pieces the images becomes less clear and quality suffers even though the full image is still there.

The concept of the person and their energy system as a holographic model reflects the idea that every part of the person has knowledge and understanding of every other part. Even though the practitioner may be focussing on a specific part of the physical body, this is not all that is being considered – the whole person is represented there.

Practitioners who use a holographic model in their work see everything as interconnected. They believe that it is not usually possible to have a simple linear cause and effect, where the cause happens and the effect is inevitably produced. Using the holographic model, the practitioner uses muscle testing to find the pieces - from that person's history, from different body systems, from different subtle bodies (see page 08), etc. - that represent the individual's dynamic needs, bringing them together in a way that gives clarity and allows insight at a deep level as to what is needed for profound and lasting healing.

In some kinesiology systems a specific finger mode (see page 21) may be used to indicate that the session is using a holographic model. This will be placed in circuit (see page 20) ahead of anything else.

Therapy Location

Therapy locating is a technique used to identify the most appropriate correction procedure to use. There are particular points connected with each of the different correction procedures for each of the meridians. Once a muscle is found that unlocks, the kinesiologist touches each of the points in turn while testing the same muscle. When the previously unlocked muscle locks that indicates the points or technique that should be used for the correcting process. Many kinesiologists use other methods of establishing what technique to use either as well or instead of therapy locating.

Priority

Many kinesiology systems work with the concept of priority. There may be a priority for what symptom or goal is tackled first. Priority is established using finger modes (see page 21) or asking verbal questions. Priority does not equal importance. Small things may need fixing before big things. For example, the energy system may want to fix a minor physical problem first, because it is getting worse rapidly, rather than a bigger problem that is chronic and debilitating but not deteriorating.

Once the priority symptom or goal is established, there may also be priority for the order of the techniques and procedures. The meridian or correction that takes priority is simply the first thing that is required. If you think about making a cake, getting the bowls out of the cupboard is not necessarily the most important thing to do, but it is one of the first.

Stress

Stress is a central concept for most kinesiologies, but the word is usually used in a broad context to include not only psychological stress but many other types of stress (e.g. allergies, nutritional imbalances, problems with hand-eye co-ordination, postural misalignment, etc.) Many kinesiologists use the analogy of a bucket: each stress in our life increases the total load in the bucket. If we do not deal with the stress appropriately, the bucket will overflow and symptoms will appear.

The kinesiologist seeks to defuse or remove or correct the stress – different terms are used by different practitioners and kinesiology systems. Because muscle testing is used to establish the priority (see above), kinesiologists believe that whatever is stressing the system can be removed without causing further stress, and that the practitioner will only be given permission to proceed (page 26) when the person is ready to address the issue or problem.

Behavioural Barometer

The Behavioural Barometer was developed by Three In One Concepts and is described as a "road-map of behavioral patterns". The Behavioral Barometer allows the client with the help of the practitioner to access conscious, sub-conscious and deep body level emotional imbalances. It is central to the work of Three in One Concept practitioners but is also used by many other kinesiologists too. (See page 151 for a more detailed discussion of the Behavioral Barometer.)

Amygdala

Although people talk about the amygdala, there are, in fact, two. Each amygdala is located close to the hippocampus, in the frontal portion of the temporal lobe of the brain. The amygdala allows us to experience emotions and to recognise emotions in other people. The amygdala is involved in our flight or fight response to danger. Many of the alarm circuits are grouped together in the brain, and process incoming sensory danger signals, etc. The amygdala processes sets of stimuli as well as individual stimuli, giving a context to the sensory input. The amygdala plays an important role in the process in which we label something as dangerous and start to feel anxious or frightened. Many kinesiologists, (such as practitioners of Applied Physiology, Integrated Healing, AcuNeuroSync/LEAP and Professional Kinesiology Provider) work with the amygdala as the place where early emotional memories are stored. These experiences, which may happen before the child is able to understand the event in its full context, can result in emotional triggers that continue to disturb us into adulthood. Other kinesiologists also work with early emotions but without recourse to the concept of the amygdala.

Psychological Reversal

Psychological reversal occurs when muscle testing shows that the person wants to keep the problem. The concept of psychological reversal was first introduced by Roger Callahan, who developed Thought Field Therapy, but has been incorporated into may kinesiology systems.

Brain Integration

Brain integration is a central concept for some kinesiologies, such as Three In One Concepts and AcuNeuroSync/LEAP. The two hemispheres of the brain are seen to perform different functions: the left hemisphere concerned with rational processing and the right hemisphere concerned more with emotions. Many people test as having one of the hemispheres dominant. While it may be important at any given moment to have a particular hemisphere of the brain dominant, a fully functioning human being will change dominance depending on the circumstances. In addition there needs to be good integration between the two hemispheres of the brain.

The techniques used work to strengthen the non-dominant hemisphere, to integrate the functioning of the two brain hemispheres and also to improve co-ordination between hands, feet, eyes, ears and the brain. The techniques often involve the client moving their body or part of their body in a set way on a regular basis.

Although this work is particularly appropriate for people with dyslexia or learning difficulties, everyone's brain needs help to function at its maximum potential.

See also AcuNeuroSync/LEAP (page 48) for more information on this.

Switching

Superficial switching is seen as being transitory neurological confusion that happens usually only in times of stress, whereas deep level switching involves transposed hemispheres and is usually present all the time. The concept of deep level switching was introduced in the late 1980's by Hap Barhydt. Charles Krebs (see page 50) sees deep level switching as a special case of the deep switching that occurs as a survival response in the brain stem and limbic system. The two hemispheres of the brain are efficient at processing different types of information: the logic hemisphere processes sequential bits of information, whereas the gestalt brain processes global, whole picture information. Both are needed for performing most tasks and complex thinking. In deep level switching the incoming information is sent to the wrong hemisphere for processing. Deep level switching problems are seen to originate either in early childhood trauma (the most common) or to be inherited (through karma, the genes or energetically). Charles found that psychological reversal (see page 33) was often involved with this deep level switching.

Gait Testing

A surprising number of people do not walk properly. When we walk properly opposing arms and legs are co-ordinated, so left arm and right leg go forward together. Gait testing involves checking that moving the arm and leg at the same time in this way does not stress the body. Testing involves applying light pressure to the opposing arm and leg at the same time. This is usually done lying on the front and then repeated with clients lying on their backs. Arms and legs out to the side may also be tested. Particular acupuncture points are massaged and clients are often encouraged to spend time each day making exaggerated walking movements.

Primitive Reflexes/ Infant Reflexes

A new born baby has certain primitive reflexes that only last for a short time. Through repetition of these involuntary reflexes the infant gains important information about the outside world, stimulating the brain and helping it to develop as it should.

For example, a very young infant cannot support its own weight, but, nevertheless, if the sole of one foot is s placed on a flat surface the baby will move its other foot forward as though walking. Normally this and other primitive reflexes disappear. If the reflexes remain, they can inhibit learning and lead to neuro-developmental delay and poor sensory integration. This can mean the child (and later the adult) has poor posture, difficulty with balance, is over-sensitive to light or sound, has difficulty grasping things, etc. Children with this problem are often labelled dyslexic, lazy, uncommunicative, aggressive, difficult, etc.

Treatment includes regularly performing exercises that simulate these early developmental movements.

Temporomandibular Joint (TMJ)

The TMJ is the jaw joint. There are, of course, actually two – one on each side of the jaw. The most common medical condition is when the articular disc moves and then bone rubs directly on bone. This is a very painful and is not usually what is meant when kinesiologists refer to clients having TMJ problems. Kinesiologists are usually referring to an imbalance or strain in the joint. TMJ problems can have a variety of causes including poor posture, excessive clenching of the jaw, teeth grinding, or as a result of an accident or dental work. People with TMJ problems may suffer from a range of problems, including headaches, insomnia, digestive problems and hormonal disturbances.

Kinesiologists will usually work to release and realign muscles, tendon sand ligaments in the area of these joints. Kinergetics, in particular, does a lot of TMJ work in its protocols.

Ileocaecal Valve (ICV)

The ICV is a muscular valve (sphincter) between the small intestine and the large intestine. Its role is to hold the chyme in the small intestine until all the nutrients have been absorbed from the small intestine; then the valve opens to allow the chyme into the large intestine. The valve also stops faecal matter going back into the small intestine. Many kinesiologists find that testing indicates that the valve is partially open, allowing the chyme to move into the large intestine before all the nutrients are extracted and/or allowing chyme to seep back into the lower portion of the small intestine leading to toxic symptoms such as lethargy and headaches.

The ICV is tested by applying pressure either upward or downward into the area and testing an indicator muscle at the same time. Various acupuncture points and neurolymphatic points are touched, pressed or massaged to reset the ileocaecal valve.

Ionization

Everyone recognises that breathing is vitally important, but some kinesiologies look at breathing in relation to ionization. The right nostril is seen as being a chamber for positive ions and the left nostril for negative ions. The dominant breathing pattern changes from one nostril to the other about every twenty minutes. Some people habitually favour one nostril more than the other. One obvious reason for this tendency is when people have catarrh, sinus problems, rhinitis or hay fever, but it can also occur without any obvious cause.

This disparity can lead to problems of midline balance and functional imbalance between the two hemispheres of the brain. One possible result of this is dyslexia. As Bruce Dewe (page 136) says: Do you remember not being able to think straight when you had a stuffy head cold?

People with this problem are also likely to be disturbed after thunder storms, because of the rapid change in positive and negative ions during and shortly after stormy weather.

Dehydration

Many kinesiologists routinely test for adequate levels of hydration in the client at the beginning of the session, because dehydration can interfere with the accuracy of muscle testing. It is also essential for the practitioner to be sufficiently hydrated before the session starts.

Many clients are not aware that they are dehydrated - thirst or a dry mouth are the final warning signs that you are in a dehydrated state, but the consequences of that are already having a detrimental effect on the body.

Kinergetics practitioners see hydration issues as being particularly important and seek to address this with many of their clients.

Geopathic Stress/Geobiology

Geopathic comes from two Greek words: geo means 'of the earth', and pathos means 'suffering' or 'disease'. The word 'geopathic' literally means suffering or disease of the earth. Geopathic stress is the negative effect of some earth energies on human beings. If you live and work above such an area, you are likely to have difficulty staying well, and if you get sick you will find it difficult to get well. If you suffer from tiredness, headaches, irritability, miscarriages, or chronic ill health that doesn't respond to treatment, you may be suffering from geopathic stress. (See my book *Geopathic Stress & Subtle Energy* for more information on this fascinating topic.)

Not all practitioners recognise or work with these energies, but those that do will seek to neutralise or counteract these energies either themselves or by bringing in someone experienced in this field.

Correction Methods

Once imbalances have been identified, there are various rebalancing procedures that can be used. Some of these work directly on the body – touching, massaging or holding specific points or areas. Other techniques include the client taking something or doing something in the session or afterwards. The image of techniques and possibilities is phenomenal. It is impossible to cover all of these, but I have endeavoured to include the ones that you are most likely to come across.

The Original Correction Techniques

These standard techniques owe much to the origins of kinesiology within chiropractic and George Goodheart's research and insights:

- Spinal Reflex technique
- Neurolymphatic
- Neurovascular
- Meridian tracing
- Origin/ insertion
- Acupressure Holding Points

Some practitioners will try these procedures one after another until one works. They are usually tried in the order above, because it has been found that it is quicker to use the spinal reflex technique than it is to use the neurolymphatic technique, which is usually quicker than the neurovascular technique, and so on. Quite often several of the different correcting techniques will work, so it makes sense to start with the one which is usually quickest to complete.

Other practitioners use the priority finger mode (see page 21 and 32) or verbal questioning (see page 22) to determine which will be most effective.

At its simplest, once a muscle imbalance is identified the correct technique can be used to rebalance the body. The muscle is then tested again to check that the re-balance has indeed occurred.

List Scanning

Some kinesiologists work with lists. These can be lists of emotions or supplements, flower remedies (see page 41), body systems or any other list that you can think of. The kinesiologist will scan the list to find the relevant item. This is usually done by placing the finger on the list or chart and moving down it looking for an indicator muscle change or for a strong response in answer to a verbal question or statement. The practitioner might hold the priority finger mode at the same time or tap the head or use eye rotation at the same time. It could also be a diagram (e.g. of the skeletal system) rather than a list.

Spinal Reflex Technique

When the spinal reflex technique is needed, identical muscles on both sides of the body weaken when tested, but both muscles can test weak when other balancing procedures are needed.

Where the spinal reflex technique is needed, it reveals the correlation of muscle inhibition and subluxation in specific vertebrae. Chiropractors and osteopaths may use spinal manipulation, whereas kinesiology practitioners, who do not have this professional background, use a simple up and down massage of the skin over the spinal process to achieve an energy balancing effect.

Neurolymphatic Corrections

The lymph system is vitally important to health. Lymph is a clear or milky fluid that is passed around the body by the contraction of muscles as we move around. The lymph system does not have the equivalent of the heart to pump the lymph. Lymph accumulates in the spaces between cells and needs to be collected and put back into the blood system. The lymph system plays an important role in the body's immune response by taking immune cells to and from the lymph glands. It also absorbs fats from the intestine.

Neurolymphatic reflex points are mainly on the torso. These are sometimes also called Chapman's reflexes. In Touch for Health these reflex points are seen as "circuit breakers or switches that get turned off when the system is overloaded". (Touch for Health manual)

The points are rubbed to stimulate lymph flow. The points are not necessarily located near lymph glands or even the muscle that they are associated with. For example, the neurolymphatic points for the opponens pollicis longus muscle (which is in the hand) are between the 7th and 8th rib on the left side of the front of the body and also on either side of the spine on the back of the body.

These points are often tender and massaging them can be a little uncomfortable. It usually seems that the more beneficial the massage is going to be the more painful the point is initially, but fortunately the points generally become less sensitive indicating the rebalancing of the system that is taking place.

Neurovascular Corrections

Most neurovascular correction points are on the head, so are usually not near the actual muscle itself. So, for example, the pectoralis major sternal, a chest muscle related to the liver meridian has a pair of neurovascular points on the natural hairline about half an inch (about 1.25 centimetres) either side of the midline.

Most of the points are bilateral, i.e. on both sides of the head. The points are usually held for 20 to 30 seconds, but occasionally a longer time is needed. The practitioner may feel a deep pulse as these points are gently held. The pulses become synchronised as the points continue to be held.

Meridian Tracing

The meridians run in a specific direction. Meridian tracing involves putting the hand on the body or just a little off the body and tracing the route of the meridian from beginning to end to enhance energy flow. This can be used during the session or as something that the client does at home.

Origin/ Insertion Massage

This is the first correction method discovered by George Goodheart. The origin of a muscle is the end that attaches to a non-moving bone, and the insertion is the part that attaches to a moving bone. Two procedures are used: jiggling and hard heavy pressure.

Jiggling involves putting the fingers at each end of the muscle, and the ends of the muscle are wiggled back and forward. Jiggling is done to a muscle that tests weak or unlocked, and it is believed that this 'wakes up' the muscle.

Hard heavy pressure is used when a muscle has been strained or overworked. Hard heavy pressure is applied usually to the origin, but the insertion of the muscle may also be massaged. It is believed that this re-establishes "the contacts, like pinning up a wisp of hair that has gone astray". (*Touch for Health* page 57.)

Acupressure Holding Points

Each muscle has related acupressure holding points on the lower arms and legs. The kinesiologist will first hold one set of points applying very light pressure and then hold the second points, again with light pressure on the same side of the body as the muscle that is being addressed. This tonifies the muscle.

Activation And Sedation Points

Sometimes practitioners will hold specific points related to specific meridians to activate or sedate the meridian. Different points are used depending on whether the meridian is being activated or sedated.

Spindle Cell Techniques

The muscle spindles are located in the belly (centre) of the muscle. They monitor the muscle length and the rate at which that length changes. Using the thumbs to either stretch out or squeeze in the muscle spindles strengthens or weakens the muscle. This can be used to relieve cramp or as part of pre-tests (see page 25) to show that the muscle is functioning properly or to strengthen a weak muscle.

Cerebro-Spinal Fluid Reflex

The cranial bones move microscopically but sometimes become "jammed", inhibiting the flow of cerebrospinal fluid that bathes the brain and the spinal cord. The correcting procedure is simple - the skin on a specific part of the head (the sagittal suture) is gently pulled apart three or four times.

Meridian Tapping

Sometimes the beginning and ends of the meridians are tapped. This is common in corrections for phobias and substance intolerances.

Temporal Tapping

Temporal tapping is used to change negative habits (such as smoking, drinking excess alcohol, losing weight) and also to reduce involuntary processes (such as the gag reflex when having a dental examination). Temporal tapping can also be used to reinforce positive habits and affirmations.

The skull is tapped around the ears. The theory is that the nerves in this area act as a filter mechanism for sensory input. In order to survive we ignore a large part of the stimuli coming into the brain. If we analysed everything at a conscious level, we would never do anything. In general we are aware only of changes in stimuli. For example, we only become aware of the ambient temperature when it changes and we become too hot or too cold; we may notice the hum of a machine only when it stops. Kinesiologists believe that the temporal tap alerts the brain to the importance of what is about to happen and so ensures that it is not filtered out.

While the client says an appropriate statement or affirmation, the practitioner or the client taps the area around the ear using the pads of the fingers. Some practitioners will use different but related statements for the two ears, to reflect the different needs of the two brain hemispheres (see page 48).

Some practitioners also tap the skull in order to access deeper levels of information when muscle testing to find the cause of a specific problem.

Affirmations

Affirmations are positive statements about a state or goal that the client wants to achieve. Affirmations do not express a wish, but express the goal as though it is now reality. So a wish to lose weight becomes translated into a positive statement, e.g. I enjoy being at my ideal weight. Affirmations may be said during a session or given as homework. Temporal tapping (see above) is often used at the same time. Although positive, affirmations can, and often do, generate stress, so energy work may be needed.

Visualisations

Visualising positive events can have a profound effect on people. The visualisation might be done as part of the session or the client may be given a specific visualisation to be done at home.

Age Regression/Age Recession

The term used for this concept varies across the kinesiologies, but the fundamental concept is that some stresses need fixing other than in the present time. In reality we can only be at the current time, but energetically it is possible to go back to the time at which a critical event happened and reconnect with it, in order to dispel the stress associated with it.

Usually the age will be determined by testing, although it may be suggested by the client and then confirmed by testing. The client will be taken gently back to that time and then after the work brought back equally gently to the present. The Behavioural Barometer (page 151) or verbal questioning are usually used to establish the emotions or thoughts involved. The practitioner may work actively to help the client replace the old memories with new, more appropriate memories, or the client may be encouraged to work through this process silently on their own. The client is then brought back to the current time.

Metaphors

Each meridian has metaphors associated with it. Matthew Thie (the son of John Thie, the founder of Touch for Health) has described the use of metaphors in this way:

> Using the metaphors helps us to verbalize or at least think about the many possible aspects of our goals and the related imbalances. When we think about a metaphor related to an imbalance indicated by a muscle test, we often have that 'Aha!' moment of insight.
> (UK Kinesiology Conference 2001)

There are metaphors, and so questions, for each of the elements (see page 11), each meridian, and each muscle. For example, the Touch for Health Manual lists these questions for the metal element:

- Are you too hard or not hard enough on yourself or others?
- Are you too focused on adornment and appearance .....?

For the lung meridian it includes these questions among others:

- Can you breathe/speak easily?
- Do you have a free flow of fresh air and/or inspiration to nourish the various functions of your life, or are you feeling constricted, inhibited in speaking, literally or figuratively?
- Do you need to shout, cheer or even cough something up?

For the anterior serratus, a muscle associated with the lung meridian the questions include:

- Do you need to exert your power to reach your goal?
- Have you lost your voice literally or figuratively?

Exploring metaphors and these questions is particularly appropriate if testing shows that particular elements, meridians or muscles are frequently unbalanced. Sometimes when the practitioner poses the question, the client gains an immediate insight, but sometimes the practitioner and client will discuss the answers to the questions, and the client may well go on thinking about them, gaining useful insights even after the session has finished.

Emotional Stress Release

Emotional Stress Release is a powerful technique that helps to remove the emotional charge of events. The event can be something that happened in the past, something that is happening now, or some stress associated with an event that might or will happen in the future.

It may be used during a session or taught to clients so that they can use it whenever they need to in their daily lives. The client or the practitioner holds the bumps on the forehead called the frontal eminences while the client thinks about the stressful situation. If the event is particularly stressful, the client might first imagine viewing it on a television. Then once some of the extreme emotions have been removed, the client imagines him/herself in the situation and continues to hold the frontal eminences until all the stress has been removed. Sometimes the event will be tackled several times from different perspectives, and sometimes additional points are held, usually on the head.

Flower Remedies And Other Essences

The original flower remedies were developed by Dr Edward Bach - pronounced Batch, not Bark - who lived in England from 1886-1936. He was trained as a doctor and worked as a pathologist and bacteriologist, but he felt that medicine was not getting to the root of the problem. He learnt about homeopathy, and developed various important homeopathic remedies, but he was still not satisfied, and this led him to develop the Bach flower remedies.

The remedies are based on flowering plants and trees, and are designed to correct inappropriate psychological states. Bach saw a close link between psychological states and physical problems; he believed that there was:

> … a factor above the physical plane which in the ordinary course of life protects or renders susceptible any particular individual with regard to disease, of whatever nature it may be.
> (*Heal Thyself* by Edward Bach)

Bach found the remedies through intuition. Sometimes he would hold a flower in his hand and experience in his body and mind what the remedy was capable of, and sometimes he experienced deep negative emotions and would go out into the countryside searching until he found the flower that would heal these feelings.

Bach also found that if he floated the flowers in a glass bowl containing spring water in the sunshine, this healing property of the flower passed into the water. For some plants that flowered early in the year, such as holly, Bach boiled the flowers and stems to overcome the problem of the lack of sunshine. He developed 38 flower remedies and one combination remedy known as Rescue Remedy.

Since then other practitioners have developed their own remedies. They often prepare them in the same way as Edward Bach, but may use crystals, weather conditions, etc. Popular ones include Alaskan Essences, Australian Bush Flower Essences, Flower Essence Services (FES), Green Man Essences, Indigo Essences, Wild Earth Essences and my own Earth Energies.

Many kinesiologists regularly use remedies and essences either during a session or for the client to take afterwards. The remedies can be given by mouth, rubbed into the body, put on an acupuncture point or sprayed around the body or part of the body. The kinesiologist will usually use muscle testing to establish the remedy, how it is used and the frequency and length of time that is appropriate.

Aura-Soma Remedies

Aura-Soma is a system of colour therapy which was developed by Vicky Wall in the UK. In 1984 she had 'a series of re-occurring meditative visions'. Vicky was a chiropodist, a pharmacist and a herbalist. She was also blind. She put together a series of bottles with two contrasting coloured liquid layers. The layers were made from essential oils, herbs, crystal energies and coloured spring water. There are now over 100 different bottles in the original balance series, plus other combinations known as Pomanders and Quintessences.

The remedy may be chosen through muscle testing, or through the practitioner or client being drawn to a particular bottle.

The remedies can be applied to specific acupuncture points, directly to an area of the body or into the aura. There is also a light beamer pen which means that light is shone through the aura-soma remedy onto the body.

Crystals

Some practitioners make extensive use of crystals and semi-precious stones, such as carnelian, quartz, jade, sodalite, tiger's eye, etc. Each crystal type is believed to have special energy properties. So, for example, sodalite is seen as calming and clearing the mind, whereas tiger's eye is used to help the digestive system. Sometimes programmed crystals are used, where the practitioner has added extra energy qualities to the stone to help healing and/or well-being. Crystals may be used in the session or placed in the home or carried by the client.

Food

Certain foods have been found to be consistently effective at strengthening particular muscles. For example, the Touch for Health Manual recommends foods that contain calcium, vitamin E and vitamin B for the heart meridian, whereas water and foods containing vitamins A and E are some of the recommendations for the kidney meridian. Of course, we are all individual so a food that is not on the recommended list may be appropriate for some people.

Nutritional Supplements

Some kinesiologists make extensive use of nutritional supplements, whereas others hardly ever use them. Sometimes Riddler's nutritional testing points are used. These relate to specific vitamins or minerals and the practitioner will test the relevant point for a particular nutrient. Some kinesiologists will find the correct nutritional supplement to strengthen a weak muscle and then give that to the client to take on a regular basis. Other practitioners use verbal questioning to establish what remedies are appropriate and how they should be taken. Sometimes the problem is caused not by a deficiency of the nutrient in the diet but by problems of absorption. In this case many kinesiologists use other correcting procedures rather than giving the client the supplement to take.

Test Kits

Some practitioners use small vials containing actual substances, homeopathic substances or the vibrational energy pattern of foods, pollens, bacteria, hormones, etc. Test kit samples can be used to check if a particular internal or external substance causes an imbalance.

Once this has been established, the practitioner may tap or hold points on the body, or test various supplements to find one that gives a change in the indicator muscle or carry out other correcting procedures.

Auricular Exercise

This usually involves unfolding the turned over part of the ears and pulling the ear away from the ear opening. Kinesiologists have found this can be beneficial for people with dyslexia, those with neck and shoulder problems and those with co-ordination problems. This may be carried out during a session, but is particularly likely to be recommended as something to do on a regular basis.

Exercises

There are two types of exercise that can be used in sessions or given as homework. There is the normal types of exercise (which improve aerobic capacity, strength and flexibility), and there are other types of exercise, sometimes called biokinetic exercises (which enhance energy connections, co-ordination and brain function). These include sitting in a particular position, so that the limbs are placed in a particular position, or making rhythmic movements with the arms and legs, etc. Practitioners use muscle testing to decide exactly which type of exercises should be done.

Working Off the Body

Some kinesiologists, but not all, work off the body some of the time, for example, – holding their hands above the body or placing crystals above the head, etc. Kinesiologists who work in this way usually also work extensively with concepts such as auric field and energetic chords (see page 43).

Does It Work?

Obviously I would not have a written a book like this if I did not believe that kinesiology works and can make a profound difference to people's health and sense of well-being. Yet, even though I practiced kinesiology for over 20 years and taught it for more than 10 years, I still at times find myself doubting that it can work. We have been brought up to believe in science, double-blind trials and the power of drugs, so can something this simple and this bizarre work?

Many people put it down to a placebo effect. This is usually done in a dismissive way: "it's only a placebo" or "it's a mere placebo" or something similar. Accepting that it is a placebo effect, this is not something to dismiss lightly. Placebos are usually cheap, and certainly kinesiology is much cheaper than conventional medicine. Unlike drugs people do not usually experience side effects from taking placebos. I once listened to an interview with the CEO of a large drug company, and he admitted that all drugs have side effects, but the benefits of the drugs that are marketed are believed to outweigh the damage they do. People are not allergic to placebos. Allergic reactions to drugs (such as antibiotics) are a real and potentially life-threatening response by some patients. Researchers have to spend money on costly research, which may involve animal testing, to find different drugs for different conditions. The placebo mechanism works across a huge range of symptoms and people. We do not need to find different placebos for different symptom sets.

Even if we value the placebo effect for the powerful health tool it is, are kinesiology benefits down to the placebo effect? Thinking back to some of my successes, it is hard to see how some of them can be down to the placebo effect:

- The man, who only worked part-time because of severe arthritis in his knees, came to see me even though he knew "it won't work, but I'm prepared to come and pay to stop my wife and my neighbour's wife nagging at me to come and see you." Three months later he was back in full time work; this time as an area sales manager travelling thousands of miles a month in a non-automatic car. He subsequently referred lots of people to me.
- The trainee nurse with psoriasis who in a weak moment let her mum make an appointment for her with me. On the day of the appointment they had a huge row, because she had decided she did not want to come and see me. They argued so badly that they drove down to my clinic in separate cars. A few weeks later the psoriasis was virtually gone in spite of the stress of looming final nursing exams. She came to her appointment bringing me a big bunch of flowers by way of apology and thanks.
- A man with macular degeneration of the eyes said at the end of his final appointment: "I don't mean to be rude. What you do is a joke, but I have no other explanation for why my eyesight is getting better."
- A bank manager who came to see me in desperation because he had bitten his nails all his life. Within a week he had stopped, although he could not make sense of what had happened in the session.

- I had a friend who was a nurse who had a frozen shoulder. I persuaded her to let me have a look at it and ended up holding acupuncture points on her knee. While I was doing this, she scoffed at me: "That's not where my shoulder is! I'm glad I don't have to rely on you!" I saw her the next day and she told me that her shoulder was much much better. She was completely amazed.
- The numerous clients who came back for a second session saying something like this: "I left after the first session and felt I'd just wasted my money. How could what you do work? I still don't understand how it works, but it did."

Incidents like this make no sense from a scientific point of view, but the level of her scepticism makes it difficult to dismiss as all down to the placebo effect. Equally animals and small babies often respond well to kinesiology, and it is difficult to see how the placebo affect would work, particularly for animals:

- One of the youngest clients I ever had was a baby who was 6 weeks old and was failing to thrive. In fact, she was losing weight because she was sick every time she was fed. Different feeds had been tried but without any success. The baby was brought to see me. She slept through the whole session, during which I established that she was reacting to the tap water that was used to mix the feed. This problem was quickly solved; the baby stopped being sick and started to gain weight much to everyone's relief.
- The dog who did not like to go for a walk started leaping around at the sound of its lead being picked up after a Health Kinesiology treatment.
- My friend's cat was a very untidy eater, scattering food everywhere – a very unusual problem to face a cat owner. A quick kinesiology session while I was visiting fixed this problem immediately.

Most kinesiologists will be able to recount similar stories. None of these cases shout *placebo*, although I do believe that the placebo mechanism was probably at work in some of the cases, but not in the sense that critics use to dismiss it, but in the sense that kinesiology is able to trigger the same mechanisms as the ones that cause the placebo effect within the person to bring about effective and lasting healing. Many kinesiologists would disagree with this, so what I am writing here is defnitely a personal view.

What should not be in dispute is that kinesiology works – not all the time and not for everyone, but when it does work it can bring about spectacular results, improving and changing people's lives for the better.

Different Kinesiology Systems

The information in this section of the book is designed to help potential clients find the right type of kinesiology and for potential kinesiologists to recognise the best kinesiology for them to study. It may also give established kinesiology practitioners some insights into the concepts and practices they share and also the ones that make their kinesiology system unique.

There is information on different systems of kinesiology. Kinesiologies represented here range from small systems developed by a single person and practiced in only one country to large organisations that have many practitioners and clients in many countries around the world. At the end of the book there are contact addresses for professional organisations and training institutes.

some kinesiology training builds on the basic muscle testing skills taught in Touch for Health courses, whereas others include teaching this fundamental skill within their system.

Some kinesiology systems have a relatively fixed protocol, feeling this is the best way to ensure that nothing is overlooked or missed, whereas others concentrate on going with the flow, feeling this allows the client's true needs to show through more clearly. Some kinesiologists will deal with specific symptoms as presented by the client, although they almost certainly will not be prepared to give a medical diagnosis (unless they have other medical training as well). Other kinesiologists will focus on generally rebalancing the body, on the understanding that this will lead to effective healing and repair. Some kinesiologies emphasise the physical body more, some focus more on subtle energies. Some kinesiologies have concepts such as higher self and soul as central to their work. There are kinesiologies where the practitioner is, respectfully, in charge, and others were the practitioner and client are seen as more like equal partners in the process.

This disparity between the different kinesiologies may at first seem disconcerting, but in many ways it can also be seen as a strength of kinesiology. Practitioners with different styles, different experiences and different interests can bring all this to the work they do, enhancing its effectiveness through the amazing tool of muscle testing. Even within a particular kinesiology system, different practitioners will focus on different aspects of their kinesiology. Of course, some practitioners will be trained in and use more than one kinesiology system and will chose whatever is appropriate at the time. Potential clients can also find the right kinesiology and right practitioner that resonates with where they are and where they want to be.

As well as descriptions of different kinesiology systems, there are interviews, case studies and pieces written by practitioners/teachers about the particular kinesiology they love.

Many kinesiologists have other professional qualifications. This is always true of diplomates of the International College of Applied Kinesiology, who are medical doctors, dentists, chiropractors, osteopaths, etc. Other kinesiology practitioners will often have qualification in other therapies such as NLP, massage, reflexology, etc. They may use these within a kinesiology setting, either in making a clinical judgement or using muscle testing to establish when a particular therapy is appropriate.

There are also practitioners whose primary therapy is not kinesiology, but who use muscle testing to support their main therapy or therapies. For example, an aromatherapist might use muscle testing to establish precisely the best oil or combination of oils for a massage treatment. Some therapists will test the whole range of oils they have at their disposal, and other therapists will only use kinesiology testing when they feel that several oils are clinically indicated, but there is no one obvious over-riding reason to choose one particular oil rather than another. A homeopath may use muscle testing in a similar way to choose between several equally indicated remedies or to establish the best potency for a particular client. Chiropractors that do not use the full AK protocols, may use muscle testing in a more limited way, for example, to confirm their diagnosis as to the exact location for an intervention procedure.

This section does not cover every kinesiology system, and omission should not be taken to imply that a particular kinesiology system is unimportant or without value. From my own training I know more about some kinesiologies than others. For those I know less about I have had to rely on studying training manuals and/or talking to teachers and practitioners. Some kinesiology systems seem to have an abundance of people who wanted to communicate with me and help me understand about their kinesiology, whereas for others I found it difficult to make any useful contacts.

AcuNeuroSync/LEAP

LEAP (Learning Enhancement Acupressure Program) was developed by Dr Charles Krebs, who was an Associate Professor of Biology at the University of Maryland, USA before moving to Australia. He became interested in kinesiology in his search for help for himself following a serious diving accident that left him in a wheelchair paralysed from the waist down. His remarkable recovery inspired him to learn more about kinesiology and develop his own system. By the beginning of 1985 he had developed a system of kinesiology to treat children with learning problems. From the early 1990's he continued to develop this work with the assistance of Susan McCrossin and named it the Learning Enhancement Acupressure Program or LEAP. He and Susan initially practiced LEAP in their clinic and were able to resolve many types of learning problems. Within a few years they began to teach this work to others both in Australia and overseas, and in the late 1990s, Susan took this work to the US and named it the Brain Integration Technique or BIT (Crossinology® Brain Integration Technique, see page 77).

Brains are designed to learn, not only when we are babies and children, although that is when learning most obviously happens, but throughout our lives. Some people are able to learn easily but others have problems mastering even basic skills such as reading and writing. Sometimes this is because of low intelligence or physical damage to the brain, but in the great majority of cases, it is not at all obvious why the person has problems learning. Often they demonstrate normal intelligence, but cannot seem to learn to read, spell properly or do mathematics. For these people the problem is usually one of accessing particular brain functions, or being able to integrate the brain functions that they do access.

Recent scientific research has shown that thinking, learning and memory are complex activities involving widely distributed systems in many different areas of the brain. These different brain areas and their functions must be synchronised and integrated in order to work effectively. The brain will always choose the simplest most direct way of performing a task, but if the most direct route is blocked, it has to find another (less efficient) way to perform the same task.

Each compensatory pathway is not only longer, but even more importantly, is less efficient and requires more physical energy and mental effort. There may be many compensatory pathways needed to complete the task, because of numerous blockages. In this situation people may become so stressed or find it so hard that they opt out of the task and stop attempting it at all. In children this sort of behaviour is often labelled as naughty or stubborn or lazy or simply just not trying hard enough.

There are two cerebral hemispheres, popularly known as the right and left brain. Each hemisphere has its own functions and its own way of processing information. The corpus callosum provides the pathways needed to integrate the different functions of each hemisphere. It is this integration that produces our higher-level mental abilities. The right hemisphere in most people is concerned with gestalt, global thinking, looking at the whole picture, whereas the left hemisphere is concerned with analytic thinking, but both hemispheres are involved at all times in all brain activity. Each brain hemisphere brings its own unique contribution to any given task, even tasks generally considered to be, or that have been labelled solely as Left Brain (analytical) or Right Brain (gestalt) in nature.

Complex tasks require complex functioning of both hemispheres and high levels of integration through the corpus callosum. So, people have problems with learning and thinking if they cannot access a particular function, or have problems integrating the two hemispheres, which results in the dominance of one hemisphere in almost all processing.

For example, people with Attention Deficit Disorder usually have the gestalt brain dominant, and so do not reason and analyse particularly well. They may read fluently but with little understanding. They often act impulsively, are easily distracted and lack focus. They are often seen as being immature. People who are left hemisphere dominant are often clumsy and have difficulty reading and spelling. Some people have problems efficiently accessing both sides of the brain and so are easily distracted, developmentally delayed, have difficulty reading, writing, etc. These people often appear lazy, confused and lethargic.

Some people have good access to both hemispheres but have poor integration between them. They can carry out tasks that are simple, demanding activity mainly from one hemisphere, but fail miserably with complex tasks demanding co-ordination of the two hemispheres. They can appear erratic and moody, only willing to try when it is something they enjoy.

Deep Thalamic Reticular Switching can also occur. This is where the wrong type of information is sent to each brain hemisphere for processing. The logical hemisphere now gets the global, big picture information, and the gestalt brain gets the sequential, logical information. This makes carrying out complex tasks extremely difficult. Someone with this problem is likely to be labelled as slow and easily confused, and as children are often said "to be off with the fairies".

Being labelled in this way (lazy, immature, stupid, erratic, etc.) only adds to the frustration and stress that these people experience, making a vicious circle of stressful learning and living. This results also in poor self-esteem and lack of self-confidence and motivation.

Many people also suffer from marginal nutritional deficiencies, which do not lead to full-blown diseases such as scurvy, but impair functioning, including brain functioning. Decision-making can become impaired resulting in more impulsive and less considered thinking and behaviour. Under increased stress (a work deadline, an exam, work overload, relationship difficulties, etc.) the brain's demand for nutrients increases. When nutrients are in short supply, the conscious rational frontal lobe activity is just not supported by the nutrients available and "shuts down", leaving the subconscious limbic and brainstem, emotionally-oriented survival systems, in charge.

Using acupressure formatting (see page 22), he developed acupressure-based correction techniques to normalise many brain functions. Charles focussed on this aspect of kinesiology, researching and developing formats for more specific areas and specific kinesiological-based assessments needed to correct different types of learning problems. The LEAP protocol he developed releases stresses in the deep brain centres, including the limbic and brainstem survival systems, which control integration of hemisphere functions. These techniques increase access to the non-dominant hemisphere and improve integration between the two hemispheres. Techniques have also been developed to help correct more specific learning issues, such as problems with reading, spelling and maths.

Most children and adults need around 8-20 hours of treatment for the LEAP Program, depending upon the exact nature of their learning problems. This can be carried out over a few days, or spread out over several weeks or months. The initial assessment of the problem uses muscle monitoring to assess functional integration and also standard tests that assess specific functions underlying academic performance, e.g. digit span, a measure of auditory short-term memory. The assessment points to what needs attention and also sets the standard by which the subsequent work can be judged. LEAP practitioners use finger modes (see page 21), formatting (see page 22) and pause lock (see page 20).

The corrections use primarily acupressure, age recession (see page 39), Emotional Stress Release, sound and light therapy. Clients are also given physical exercises to do at home to help maintain brain integration. Practitioners may also recommend nutritional supplements that have been developed by Charles for this specific purpose. These supplements contain vitamins, minerals, amino acids, fatty acids and memory-enhancing herbs along with homeopathic synergists. (See Charles' book *Nutrition for the Brain. Feeding your Brain for Optimum Performance*).

The original LEAP system focused on improving brain function, so that children could learn more effectively and people could find it easier to think clearly and make appropriate decisions. Application of the LEAP Protocol consistently led to improvements not only in learning, but also in self-confidence, self-image and reduced levels of stress. As the system developed, however, it became clear to Charles that the system could be applied to many other conditions than just learning enhancement. In 2011 he changed the name of the overall system to AcuNeuroSync, with an expanded set of techniques to address imbalances in the neurological, musculoskeletal, immune and hormone systems. LEAP is now the subsidiary program of AcuNeuroSync that is focussed on the brain, neurology and learning problems.

www.lydiancenter.com/practitioners/charlesKrebs.php

Dr Charles Krebs, Australia and USA, talking about AcuNeuroSync/LEAP

Like many people who find their way into complementary medicine, I had a rough route into kinesiology. I was a chief research scientist in a marine pollution monitoring unit for the state of Victoria [Australia]. I was working as an analytical chemist. I had a Ph.D in Biology and Physiology and had also studied palaeontology, population dynamics, analytical chemistry and neurology. I loved the job and the country. As many marine scientists do, I used to go scuba diving when I wasn't working. On my recreation leave I was diving off a national park, an area with beautiful clear waters and incredible underwater rock formations. There were three of us, and we had spent a week preparing for a dive to a depth of 200 feet, the limits of compressed air diving, to look for a wreck that one of my friends thought he had spotted on a previous dive.

The dive was perfect but, on the way back into the shore, I started to get symptoms of cerebral spinal bends. This means that nitrogen gas bubbles had formed inside my brain and spinal cord. As the bubbles get bigger, they block the blood flow and crush the surrounding neurons. We were on our way to have a picnic with a doctor we knew, so we radioed ahead to him. He said I needed to get help immediately, as I almost certainly had type 2 bends. He suggested I contact Bass Strait Medical Services in a nearby local town. The two GPs who ran the centre specialised in decompression sickness (the bends) because of the number of oilrig divers in the area. At that time there were only two saturation chambers in the world, and one just happened to be nearby on a huge barge that was erecting oilrigs for Esso. I was flown out to the barge and went through the standard decompression procedure, but it didn't help. I was at that point paralysed from the neck down and was diagnosed as quadriplegic.

The doctor in charge, Geoffrey McFarlane, tried everything he knew to help me, but eventually he came to me and said: "You are a quadriplegic, and it is my opinion based on over a hundred decompressions like this one that if we go to the surface now you will be a quadriplegic the rest of your life! However, this is something that has never been tried before, but in theory it may produce major improvement, or you will die!" I decided to go for it, and the treatment (although very painful) was very successful; I exited the decompression chamber a T-9 paraplegic paralyzed from the waist down. I then began a process of rehabilitation that was clearly designed to help me live in a wheelchair, as I was told I would never walk again.

I did walk again using tools that at the time I didn't even know how to name – energetic tools. I had been a martial artist for 15 years and had taught anatomy and physiology for nine years in university. I had a semi-photographic memory so I could visualise all the nerves from my motor cortex to any specific muscle in my body. I then started running Ch'i down individual nerves to a specific muscle. I did this all day, every day until I could contract that specific muscle, but not yet move my leg, but it felt like my leg again rather than someone else's leg! Once I could contract the muscle I started doing intensive physio using weights, gradually increasing the weight. After I could move 10 kilos with that muscle, I'd move on to another muscle. I spent six months doing this intensively and at the end I could walk although not well – I was dragging my feet and arching my hips, but I could walk. When I left the unit, the neurologist just shook his head and said he didn't understand how it was possible, as I was one of the most physically damaged people on that ward. He said it was a miracle – that way he didn't have to think about what it meant and what I'd done. I wore steel-plates on the tips of my shoes and used to wear them out in a month because I was dragging my feet so badly.

The medical doctors thought I should be happy with that, but I decided to try complementary therapies to see if I could walk better. I tried osteopathy, chiropractic, homeopathy, massage, faith healing, and many other different types of therapies; most helped a bit.

Then a friend called Hugh said to me: "There's a kinesiologist called Dr Bruce Dewe (see page 136) over from New Zealand, and he does kinesiology and I think it might help! I've made an appointment for you to see him next Wednesday at 2 o'clock. Can you make it?" I could, so I decided to go, but it was one of the flakiest things you could imagine – he wiggled the hyoid bone in my neck, when I had problems with my legs! I watched my arm go up and down, when he said things and touched different points on my body. It seemed mystical, but at the end I got up, and I found my whole neurology had been reorganised. This isn't possible, not two and a half years after an accident – any medical person can tell you that. I walked out with my cane in my hand and with a much more normal gait, no longer dragging my feet.

51

That was Wednesday; on the Friday I was in my first kinesiology course with Bruce. I wanted to find out what had happened to me. The course was good, but it did not answer some of the questions I had. While I had extensive knowledge about neural physiology, I knew nothing about kinesiology or energy medicine, so this stuff was just plain weird, but it did work. I needed to know how!

One of the things I struggled with after my first kinesiology course was: if this innate wisdom or the "body" knows what the problem is and knows how to affect it, why doesn't it fix it? At the time I was seeing an acupuncturist who'd been a Zen Buddhist monk for part of his life. We'd often talk after my session, so I asked him this question. He said I was correct, but the part of the body that knows how to fix it is not directly connected to the part that has the problem – this is the role of the therapist – to connect them.

I kept on doing more and more courses and reading about subtle energy. After the diving accident I had one a half years off work. Then I returned to work as Chief Analytical Chemist and Head of the Victoria State EPA Water Quality Laboratory. It was like yin and yang ; I didn't feel comfortable at first talking to people in the lab about kinesiology.

One of my staff suffered with bad headaches, and one day she came into my office, her eyes glassy with pain. She said she had a headache and needed to go home. So I decided to take a chance and told her I did this unusual acupressure stuff with kinesiology and might be able to help. It worked. After that she would come up to me with her arm outstretched and say: "Fix my headache." Eventually I persuaded her to let me do a proper session, so that we could look at the issues underneath that caused her headaches. She'd been having headaches 3-5 times a week for fifteen years, but in the following year she had one headache, and that was caused by too much red wine!

I was totally fascinated by kinesiology and began to work evenings and weekends in a clinic as well as at my full time job as head of the lab.

I've always been lucky and been able to follow my heart in what I do. At one time I was passionate about sport and good at it. I loved studying, teaching, and research, and had gotten my Ph.D., had been teaching in university for nine years and I was a successful research scientist. I was a born research scientist with an insatiable curiosity about why and how things worked especially plants and animals. I've been a scientist since I was nine years old, when I investigated why ants follow each other in lines and discovered that they lay down chemical trails. But now I was at a point where there were two paths with heart – research science or healing - which was I going to do? In the end I resigned my position at the lab and went to America to study with Richard Utt (see page 63). Then I went back to Australia to start my full-time clinical practice.

I'd always been interested in why some people learn easily and some people don't. I have friends who I thought were intelligent, but they had so many problems with basic functions such as reading and spelling. I got interested in how kinesiology could help them. At the time I was teaching speed reading part time, and in the breaks and before and after class I was always pushing on someone's arm and performing various tests. I started testing people against two symbols: X and two parallel lines (‖). It's a coarse, but very effective way of testing visual integration – how the two eyes work together to take in coherent visual information.

People who were strong on X and inhibited on ‖ had a reading speed of around 250 words a minute; they read each word individually and so had poor comprehension overall. People who were strong on X and ‖ read at about 400 to 500 words a minute; they had peripheral and focussed integration and read three to five words at a time, which meant they could easily understand what they read. People who were weak on X and strong on ‖ had no peripheral focus and couldn't integrate on the midline. Reading was very stressful for them and they had poor concentration. They averaged 175 to 200 words a minute. The kinesiology testing was totally predictive - it proved to be a reliable predictor of people's actual objective performance as measured on standard reading tests. I worked with all sorts of people from school children to lawyers; it made no difference - I saw the same results all the time.

I had continued to take every kinesiology course I could find, always trying to understand in greater depth what had happened to me. Applied Physiology was soon the main focus of my clinical practice, as it was based in the anatomy and physiology I knew so well and made the most sense to me. However, several of the other course programs I studied purported to assist children and adults with learning problems. Indeed, I did see changes in people's learning after applying these techniques, often with remarkable improvements in reading, reading comprehension, spelling and math.

I then made a synthesis of all the different techniques that I had learnt and put them together in a structured programme that I called LEAP – the Learning Enhancement Acupressure Program. I was then asked to present my work to a group of five clinical psychologists by the director of the Speed Reading centre where I was still teaching part-time. Four said: "Interesting, goodbye", but the fifth said that what I had said made sense. She said she wanted to send me her basket cases, and if I could change them at all she would consider my work a success. She sent me a child with all sorts of problems and was amazed at the results, saying: "The boy you sent back to me is not the boy I sent to you based on unheard of changes in his scores on standard psychometric tests." She then began to send me a lot more kids.

I was now seeing very difficult cases of children for whom other remedial techniques had not worked, sent to me by the clinical psychologist as a port of last hope, but the techniques I'd learnt were only successful some of the time.

As a research scientist this bothered me. Why could these techniques be so successful, even spectacularly so, often, but fail to help others with what appeared similar problems? I then went back to first principle reasoning about how the brain must work to produce these results. I developed a model of brain function which had no direct scientific support at the time, 1985, but has since been shown indeed to be how the brain does work. I have continued to expand, revise and modify the original theory in the light of new neurological discoveries.

Because of my training in science and neurology I could talk to speech therapists, doctors, psychologists, neurologists – while I did what appeared to them to be weird "stuff", I had the language to talk to them. I trained an associate, who then became my wife Susan [McCrossin], to do the LEAP programme, and she joined me full time in my clinical practice. Although very bright, Susan had struggled in school. Following her own brain integration, Susan went to university and did a double degree in Neuroscience and Psychology, with Honours. She then took the original LEAP programme to the USA and named it BIT (see page 77).

All the time LEAP was developing – but not from me sitting down and just thinking about things theoretically – I was solving problems in the clinic, working with these super hard cases referred to me. It was very engaging for me – I love solving problems. Neurology was exploding – every year there was new information about how the brain worked, and in the past five years there has been a substantial paradigm shift of some type in this knowledge. I have been able to turn these new understandings into a new application for successfully treating previously intractable neurology problems.

I feel so blessed. Every day I go into the clinic and know I'm going to be part of some incredible experience in someone's life. I get just as excited as when I started twenty-five years ago. Every day and every person is unique. You never know what you are going to do – every treatment is a mystery tour. I get bored easily, but how can I get bored with this?

LEAP started out as what the name says – about enhancing learning, but my practice is more varied than that. I help people with immune imbalances, hormonal imbalances, psycho-emotional problems, and structural and muscular problems.

I like working with athletes and have worked with professional cricketers and principal dancers with the Melbourne ballet. In the mid-1990s I was offered a contract with the Australian Sports Institute. It would have been so much fun, so rewarding and so profitable, but what are a few points on one person's personal best compared with a child's ability to learn? You change the whole life for a child who can't read, can't do math and now can - after following the LEAP program.

Kinesiology is a tool and the other knowledge gives you a context to use that tool. I have currently stopped teaching LEAP in the workshop format, as you need an in-depth knowledge of neurology in order to use it effectively. It's not a simple form of kinesiology. The simpler forms of kinesiology may only require several weekend workshops to provide valuable skills and resolve many types of problems, and thus are valuable; but LEAP needs an extended integrated training to be used effectively.

In the beginning I offered LEAP as a series of workshops but it was just too complex to teach in this format, and I was not able to provide the ancillary supporting knowledge in anatomy and physiology and energy systems of the body, so only relatively few people were able to use it to its fullest potential. To fully use LEAP, the training must include not only kinesiology, but also the basic anatomy and physiology underlying the neuro-anatomy and neuro-physiology upon which LEAP is built. You also need an in-depth understanding of the energy systems of the body and how they may be applied to re-synchronise neurological function.

It is currently taught in longer courses with in-depth study of the energy systems of the body and neurology and assessment to demonstrate proficiency in Germany and Austria. In the US I am setting up programs to teach people who have a professional background and a license to touch.

The LEAP techniques continued to develop as I applied my wide-ranging knowledge of anatomy and physiology and neurology to many other types of imbalances and problems, many seemingly unrelated to learning problems. I am now in the process of changing the name of this whole body of techniques as the term LEAP with its emphasis on learning has become problematic. The new name is AcuNeuroSync with LEAP being but one component of AcuNeuroSync - the component that deals with correcting learning problems.

Kinesiology in general, and AcuNeuroSync in particular, has a ridiculously broad scope compared to the more specialised divisions practiced in Western medicine. AcuNeuroSync techniques can be applied to imbalances and problems that would be treated with a variety of traditional Western techniques such as occupational therapy, physiotherapy, developmental optometry, psychology and various medical procedures. It's truly multi-dimensional in its application and effect for two reasons. Firstly, it deals with the whole being, from the physiological, physical, psychological, mental to even spiritual levels, and, secondly, it uses the most effective bio-feedback tool I know – muscle monitoring or kinesiology. It is effective at every level of our being, because of the interface between the muscles and energy systems of the body and the subconscious and even unconscious systems of the body. The use of direct muscle biofeedback provides the keys to the kingdom of our being – in this it is truly remarkable.

After my accident I spent twelve years reading the Eastern scientific literature about the chakra-nadi system and the acupuncture meridian system and the rules and principles by which they work. With my extensive knowledge of neurology, I have been able to construct a cogent, coherent model of how muscle monitoring works at a neuro-physiological level and how it interfaces with the energy systems of the body. Muscle responses cannot only inform us of imbalances within our skeletal-muscular systems, but also within the energetic systems of the body as well.

My life is dedicated to getting this work out to as many people who need it as possible, and also to doing research to validate its effectiveness so that it may take its place in mainstream therapies, and be more widely available to assist people to achieve their true potential. But to do so I will need to find money in order to fund this research. I conducted a controlled research study with a PhD student in Israel, and the results were highly statistically significant (at the 0.001 level indicating that they were highly unlikely to have happened by chance). However, we cannot get this research published in traditional scientific journals, because it's based on a technique called acupressure formatting (see page 22), and the scientific research to show how that basic technique works has yet to be done. It can be so frustrating to have developed an effective technique to resolve in large part such a pressing problem as learning difficulties, but then not be able to bring it into the mainstream because of lack of evidence of its efficacy! I am constantly told: "We will believe you, when you show us the data," but then: "Oh no, we will not give you any money for research, because after all, it is an unproven technique."

I have thought a lot about my accident. There was no good physiological explanation of why I had the accident - three of us made a well-planned dive, the other two were fine and I was totally bent and almost died. This makes you think about free will and predestination. I think that certain things are set in life; they're predestined - set by the soul - experiences you have to have. But what you do with them, what the personality does with what happens to you - that's where free will operates.

I have had a challenging life. I'm now 65 and have a highly compensated body because of the diving accident. I still live in relatively high levels of pain every day all day, but I can transcend the pain; that is, I have pain and no suffering. Pain is only a nerve signal like every

55

other nerve signal, just an uncomfortable one. If you just acknowledge it hurts, but do not let your mind get hold of pain, you do not suffer, but I do face the challenge of living in an increasingly disabled body. I don't know how much time I have left to actively pursue this goal, but I'm devoting the rest of my life to getting the research done in order to get this work into the mainstream and to continue to develop new techniques to permit people to have less painful and more fulfilling lives.

I am also currently writing a textbook, The Fundamentals of Energetic Kinesiology, to raise the credibility of the work we do. I have the research skills but it takes money. I recently moved to the US, even though I would prefer to live in Australia, but I want to get the research moving and develop a professional training program to replace myself many times over, and this is the place I need to be to make this happen. It's my sacrifice to develop this work that helps so many; it's the very centre of my life; I feel it is the purpose for me still being here.

Charles Krebs, PhD, Cambridge, Massachusetts, USA
www.lydiancenter.com/practitioners/charlesKrebs.php

Applied Kinesiology

Applied kinesiology was developed by George Goodheart (see page 03) for chiropractors and others who are licensed to diagnose. Because of this, it is probably the kinesiology system that is most closely allied to the medical model.

Some practitioners say they do applied kinesiology even though they are not diplomates of the International College Of Applied Kinesiology. In general they are not meaning to deceive but are using the term applied kinesiology as a general term covering all kinesiologies that are not the academic type.

Applied Kinesiologists often make extensive use of the Triad of Health (see page 31), focussing on structural, biochemical/nutritional and mental aspects of the person. Treatment can include holding or rubbing precise points on the body, structural manipulation (if the diplomate has the necessary skills and qualifications), nutritional supplements and counselling.

The section on the history and origins of kinesiology has more information about this important discipline.

www.icak.com

Dr Clive Lindley-Jones, UK, talks about Applied Kinesiology

My original training was in the social sciences and after a few years traveling the world, I did teach sociology briefly, but, while I enjoyed teaching and have carried on doing so over my career, I was not happy changing the world through theory and wanted something more concrete and human. This is what led me to become an osteopath.

I qualified in 1981 when I was in my mid-thirties. I was originally attracted to the classical Sutherland approach to cranial osteopathy and went on a number of post-graduate courses in the early 80's. I went on one that focused on the TMJ (see page 34). At that course I saw David Walther's second AK volume on the stomatognathic system. I was impressed by the scholarship and the accuracy of the illustrations. I wasn't the only one; a few of us started to get excited about it. In the early 1980's the only ICAK diplomate in Europe was Richard Meldener DC in Paris, so we invited him to come and teach us. He came over for several years in the summer and would teach various AK modules. So Richard became my first AK teacher.

It was incredibly exciting and enormously frustrating - I had a vision of what was possible but was awash in a rather confusing tsunami of techniques and ideas. I found it difficult to fully make sense of it at this stage. Then fellow AK student Chris Astill-Smith managed to pass the diplomate exams. At the time this seemed miraculous - that anyone could make sense of all this stimulating but confusing information.

You have to remember that at that time the US seemed a long way away, and there was no world wide web. In the summer of 1889 the annual international ICAK Conference was held in London, and George Goodheart (see page 03) and David Walther were invited to speak. After that Chris Astill-Smith started to teach the ICAK 100-hour basic course. One day he suggested I attended the course to see if there was more for me to learn. I decided to continue and do the whole course through and went back for more, until Chris encouraged me to study for the diplomate exams, and eventually I went to Brussels and Detroit to sit the exams in 1992.

 After that I gave up regular undergraduate teaching so that I could began to teach the basic AK courses. I taught the standard ICAK courses for some years; I also taught specialist courses on AK & Nerve Entrapment and other AK means of unscrambling difficult problems that I have developed from the collected wisdom of AK. Over the years I have enjoyed teaching around Europe. I also teamed up with my long term AK enthusiast, osteopath Mark Mathews and helped him develop the Sunflower Trust, (www.sunflowertrust.com), using our AK skills to help children with learning difficulties such as dyslexia.

One of the things I like about AK is that you meet and become friends with professionals outside your own sphere, so old animosities between, say, chiropractors, medics and osteopaths disappear. We all have in common a fascination with this extra diagnostic tool that George Goodheart developed and shaped. For me another of the great appeals of AK has been both the inter-professional, and international nature of AK.

The way that AK is developing is particularly exciting in the German-speaking world. For example, I have just come back from attending the International ICAK meeting in Berlin where there were 350 osteopaths, medical doctors, chiropractors, dentists, physiotherapists and academic researchers from 17 countries, all with the common love and interest in AK, sharing all sorts of interesting research covering both internal medicine, manual medicine and dentistry.

It is a sad reflection on the far narrower, less informed climate of medical thinking in the UK that such a large and stimulating group of varied health professionals would be unlikely to come together. Outside of the minority of osteopaths, chiropractors and handful of dentists and doctors who are interested in AK, there are few enlightened clinicians in the UK who take seriously the wonderful tool that is AK. It seems difficult to incorporate these ideas within the largely state-controlled medical practice in England. In Germany and Austria AK has been incorporated as an advanced elective course for doctors to study. There is no reason it shouldn't happen in England, but there is, sadly, little interest. AK, more often, is regarded with suspicion or even derision, borne out of ignorance.

People sometimes ask me when I use osteopathy and when I use AK. This seems a strange question to me. AK is primarily a diagnostic tool that allows me to apply osteopathy and functional medicine with greater accuracy and precision. It's a perfect fit – adding manual muscle testing to all the other diagnostic tools and tests. I see manual muscle testing as another means of accessing the wisdom of the body. There's one caveat: if you're not careful, you can make all sorts of stupid mistakes - you have to be accurate, knowledgeable and precise. As George Goodheart said: "The body doesn't lie." But a poor grasp of AK, like anything else, poorly applied, can equally produce the garbage in garbage out situation.

AK is what it is; there are advantages and limitations, but it's a wonderful tool. I have seen it help so many people in the last twenty five years.

Clive Lindley-Jones, Oxford, UK
www.helixhouse.co.uk

Applied Kinesiology: Dr Bonny Liakos, USA, Case Study

Melinda (not her real name) was 51 years old when she came to see me. She was complaining of severe eczema covering her face, neck, anterior and posterior torso, her buttocks, thighs and upper arm regions. Melinda informed me that she had been seeking help for this condition over the past six years. She stated that she had been treated by allopathic doctors, nutritionists, chiropractors, naturopaths and other alternative health care providers, but had only minimal improvement.

Her other symptoms were extreme fatigue, digestive problems, memory issues and hearing loss. After a comprehensive examination and case history, I determined that she was suffering from a combination of different immune suppressing conditions.

Foremost was a severe case of 'Candida'. She also exhibited sensitivity to heavy chemicals, heavy metal accumulation, electro-magnetic field problems, and a toxic overload of 5 out of 5.

The first protocol I put her on was a food sensitivity/Candida/mold program. This consisted of testing her on over 200 foods and chemicals, as well as 75 different molds and several strains of Candida. After testing everything, I put her on several products (homeopathic as well as nutritional) to help her body rid itself of her food sensitivities and Candida/mold problems. She was also put on a special diet where her food and chemical sensitivities were avoided, along with sugar, yeast products and fermented foods. She was then desensitized through the brain using a special laser which allowed the brain to heal her leaky gut syndrome, flip the pH of her large intestine back to normal and get rid of her food sensitivities and Candida/molds. The nutrients/homeopathy and diet were utilized to aid the brain to make these changes permanent within a three week period of time.

Besides the Candida/mold protocol, I corrected Melinda's cranial imbalances, rebalanced her muscular skeletal system, removed subluxations, corrected her gait issue and used several other techniques to re-balance the structure, biochemistry and brain aspects within the triad of health.
At the end of this three week period of time, her eczema had diminished 75%. All of her digestive problems had been resolved. Melinda told me she was thinking more clearly and had more energy than she had had in years. In regard to her hearing loss, she informed me that this was a familial problem, but we were both hopeful we could prevent it from worsening.

The next protocol she was put on was to remove the heavy metals, correct the electro-magnetic field imbalance and get rid of her heavy chemical sensitivities. Once again she was tested on all the heavy metals, checked and corrected for lymphatic blocks, leaky fillings and a re-balancing of electro-magnetic meridian pathways. Melinda was then tested on over 50

59

heavy chemicals as well. Using the same laser and technique, I desensitized her through the brain to all of the things she had tested positive for and put her on appropriate nutrients and homeopathy. She was instructed to take three baths a week in the Masada Dead Sea salts, exercise to perspire, drink only filtered or distilled water and avoid all products containing the heavy metals and chemicals she was sensitive to.

Once again all structural imbalances were corrected: from cranial involvement to blocks in neuro-lymphatic and vascular systems. AK biofeedback was also utilized, along with several other techniques. At the end of the six week period of time Melinda was 100% eczema free. She told me that she had not felt this well in over twenty years. She was ready to start living her life again. The toxic load was now a 1 out of 5, and she told me that she believed she was hearing a little better than she had prior to starting her treatment with me. Although no official hearing tests were performed on this patient, her improvement in hearing was attributed to a reduction in inflammation within her inner ear.

When a patient comes in exhibiting many immune suppressing conditions and severe toxic overload, it is very important to correct these problems and then help the body rebuild itself. I have found in over 26 years of practice that it is incorporating the brain into the scenario that actually helps the body heal and get well. The need for dietary change, nutrients, homeopathy and structural correction play a very important role in allowing the brain to make the corrections necessary to help a patient achieve their optimal health potential.

Bonnie Liakos. New York, USA
www.drliakos.com

Applied Kinesiology: Dr Carl T. Amodio, USA, Case Study

Carrie, not her real name, came to my office complaining of feeling light-headed, having shortness of breath and mood swings. Additional questioning revealed she was also experiencing arthritic pain, back pain, chest pain, fatigue, headaches, menstrual cramps, neck pain, numbness, and dizziness.

A patient presenting with these symptoms should immediately receive further examination and differential diagnosis in order to rule out potential pathologies or life threatening conditions. After I had determined that the patient's complaints were not life threatening, further examination and treatment options were pursued.

The patient was initially examined using a combination of orthopedic tests, postural analysis, cerebellar testing, palpation, and muscle testing. Hair analysis was also undertaken to check for heavy metal toxicity, which would be causing added stress on the immune system. This showed that she had toxic levels of mercury and aluminum. Additionally, an evaluation of her hormonal status was obtained with a saliva hormone test that demonstrated too little estradiol and testosterone for a premenopausal woman.

It was apparent from our initial consultation and examination that she was suffering from significantly disturbed functional biomechanics and also disturbed functional biochemistry.

Postural analysis revealed an elevated left ilium (pelvic bone) and an elevated left scapula (shoulder blade). Subluxations were identified at various places along the spine. Muscle testing demonstrated that there were also problems with the left gluteus medius, left psoas, both sartorius, and both gracilis. All subluxations were corrected with specific chiropractic adjustments.

The patient performed the one-leg Romberg's test with eyes open and eyes closed. This single-leg test showed a stable leg stance for 20 seconds for each leg with eyes open. With eyes closed it was 15 seconds on the left leg and 5 seconds on the right leg. Palpation tenderness was noted at the level of various vertebrae and the left ilium. Carrie generally had poor posture and some limitation in her movements.

Neurolymphatic reflexes associated with inhibited muscles were stimulated with gentle but firm rotary massage for approximately 60-90 seconds each. Adrenal, ovary, and thyroid neurolymphatics were treated.

The TMJ dysfunction (see page 34) was addressed in order to restore proper muscle spindle cell activity and unlock the encoded trauma in the area. The immune system was driving the TMJ dysfunction due to overall stress precipitated by adrenal dysfunction. The adrenal challenge test was performed and addressed on the second visit and checked each visit subsequently. The immune circuits were also addressed on most of the visits and needed to be reset and strengthened frequently with nutritional supplementation and neurolymphatic work.

An aspirin mix (Aspirin/Acetaminophen/ Ibuprofen), was orally tested with muscle testing. This indicated excessive systemic inflammatory responses. Fish oil was then orally tested and indicated at this point. In addition, an antihistamine mix (Yakitron, Cimetidine, and Diphenhydramine) was orally tested with an inhibited muscle and showed a strengthening response. This indicated excessive histamine and a systemic allergic reaction. The allergies were then treated by injury recall technique.

Recommendations were made regarding dietary changes and exercise. I also recommended nutritional supplements to help reduce inflammation, encourage tissue healing and to support the endocrine and immune systems.

Carrie responded favorably to the initial therapeutic intervention. The light-headedness, shortness of breath, and mood swings disappeared after the first visit. Subsequent testing at the second visit showed she now also had an increased range of motion, improved cerebellar tests and functional improvement in muscle strength. A progressive and continual alleviation of all symptoms occurred with subsequent visits, so that at the end of three months and eleven consultations she was symptom free.

The protocol that was followed looked to clear the underlying systemic factors, to allow for more permanent and lasting corrections of the more local complaints and issues.

Carl T. Amodio, DC, Roswell, Georgia, USA
www.wholebodyhealth.org

This account is based on a case study first published in *The International Journal of Applied Kinesiology and Kinesiologic Medicine*.

Applied Kinesiology: Dr Paul T. Sprieser, USA, Case Study

Karen (not her real name) was a 17 year-old female who had a history of episodic paroxysmal vertigo that started in early childhood at 13 ½ months old when she could finally push herself into a sitting position; she didn't crawl until 16 months of age. For the first six years of her life she had had episodes of vertigo and vomiting occurring about once every month. They varied in duration from four hours to 30-40 hours. They usually began in the early hours of the morning during sleep. After this Karen continued to have episodes of vertigo lasting perhaps 30 hours and occurring every 2-3 months.

Her symptoms at the time of the initial consultation and examination were intense illusions of rotation of the environment towards the left, associated nausea, profuse vomiting, and diaphoresis (excessive sweating). The reoccurrence of symptoms had forced her to drop out of her senior year of high school and do home studies.

Her symptoms seem to be time related. She stated that the vertigo would usually wake her up between 5 am to 7 am and continue till 3:00 pm and stop abruptly.

On the first visit a standard physical examination was performed, and the only remarkable findings were limited lateral flexion in the cervical spine, absence of biceps reflex on the right and left patellar reflex was +1. Her blood pressure showed 105/82 seated and 95/62 standing which represented postural hypotension (Ragland's effect).

The AK examination revealed switching, cloacal reflex right anterior inspiratory, righting reflex right inspiratory, cranial fault-bilateral inspiratory assist, Pelvic category #1 Rt. PI, Fixations C1 Rt. Posterior, Transitional T11 right posterior, occipital side slip right, and PRYT, Pitch in flexion, Roll right, Yaw #2 on left, and Isogai (longer stride) left.

It is interesting that the vertigo starts at 6.00 am which is the time of the large intestine meridian and stops at 12.30 pm, which is heart meridian time. The treatment was tapping the heart 5 acupuncture point for sixty seconds.

The patient was clear of any symptoms of vertigo and associated nausea and vomiting for a week after the treatment but eventually she had some recurrence. After the second visit she remained symptom-free for over two months. I treated her one more time, and she remained free of vertigo for another four months. I treated her one more time and had a good response.

After this she had some treatment from a Chi Master who used Qi-Gong. She was also given some Chinese herbs and has remained clear until the present time as far as I know.

Paul T. Sprieser, D.C., Parsippany, New Jersey, USA
www.paulsprieser.com

This account is based on a case study originally published in *The Collected Paper of ICAK-USA-2001* and *The International Journal of Applied Kinesiology and Kinesiologic Medicine* 2002, issue No. 14, Fall 2002

Applied Physiology

Applied Physiology (AP) was developed by Richard Utt, an electrical engineer and expert in aeroplane flight control systems. As a young man, he was told that he should prepare to die owing to severe health issues that the doctors were unable to help. Richard did not accept this and, on a friend's recommendation, went to see an Applied Kinesiology practitioner, Dr Sheldon Deal. As Richard recovered, he studied these Applied Kinesiology techniques, as well as anatomy, physiology and neurology. He began to put it all together, and in time developed a new kinesiology modality that he called Applied Physiology.

In AP, disease is seen as being an opportunity to make changes that will enhance the client's spiritual growth, because the disease itself indicates that the person is not following physical and metaphysical laws. 'Dis-ease' within the physical body gives clues that there are also emotional, mental and spiritual imbalances that need to be addressed. Rather than the disease being fixed by an outside expert, the AP practitioner works so that individuals consciously participate in what is going on and understand what is needed to enhance their own well-being and spiritual development.

Through his extensive studies and research, Richard introduced many innovations to the field of kinesiology. He found that there are seven states of neurological muscle stress, identified through spindle cell manipulation (see page 37). This could provide important information that the practitioner could use during the session. He also introduced the concept of monitoring muscles in both contraction and extension, throughout their entire range of motion, to provide more complete neurological information. This later became the basis for Applied Physiology's 'holographic' method of assessing energy imbalances. In this system, each of fourteen positions of a muscle offers a meridian relationship to the originating muscle's meridian, providing the practitioner with a host of important and useful information.

Applied Physiology uses the pause lock system (see page 20) and hand modes, both originally introduced by an Applied Kinesiologist, Dr Alan Beardall. Combining these techniques with the use of body points (such as the alarm points of Chinese medicine), Richard established a deep method of asking complex questions of the body called formatting (see page 22). The use of formatting allowed Richard to develop new assessment methods, including specific formats to identify stressors in areas of the brain and their specific functions.

As Applied Physiology continued to evolve, Richard expanded the concept of the Chinese five element model to a seven element model. Air and ministerial fire elements are added to wood, fire, earth, metal and water, allowing integration of the more spiritual components of Chinese medicine with the physical aspects of the other five elements.

Richard researched and developed a set of 14 meridian tuning forks. These match the seven elements (see page 11) and the 14 meridians (see page 09). The tuning forks are used throughout the AP system, and can be used alone or in combination with almost any healing modality, such as flower essences (page 41), affirmations, etc. Due to the neurological basis of AP, methods of balancing that incorporate all the senses are used. Colour, hand and foot reflexology, acu-touch and acupressure may be used. Each of these is applied in a unique manner within the three-dimensional holographic method of AP.

The 7 Chi Keys, whose development was triggered by Richard's dreams, is a method of balancing the seven major chakras (see page 08) using the acupressure system. The chakras are seen as being part of the subtle energy system but also having strong links to the endocrine (hormone) and nervous systems of the body. The chakras also form a powerful link between the physical body and the subtle energy system. The AP tuning forks and special crystals are used as further balancing options. Richard considers the 7 Chi Keys to be the 'crown jewel' of his work.

Other holographic methods developed within the model of Applied Physiology include the dyslexia hologram, the cranial and TMJ (see page 34) holograms, the anatomy/physiology hologram, the Tao of blood hologram (blood chemistry), the cell hologram, and more, each with its own method of identifying related imbalances and correcting procedures.

Prior to his development of the holographic model, Richard drew from his exposure to AK, developing and expanding AK techniques and procedures. AP includes these foundational methods, such as Pitch, Roll and Yaw (PRY) and Centering, which address deep neurological and reflex imbalances that affect the body's structure and ability to function. Also, through his own research, he developed a method of working with amino acids (the building blocks of enzymes, some hormones, cellular machinery, muscles, antibodies, blood plasma, etc.). On the energetic side, Richard expanded on the traditional use of figure eights, and developed a system of working with them using the AP tuning forks that remains a central balancing method in the AP repertoire.

Richard Utt is undoubtedly the originator of many powerful and unique insights and protocols that advanced the field of kinesiology. Many of his concepts have either been taken up enthusiastically by other kinesiology systems, or led to the origination of whole new modalities.

www.appliedphysiology.com

Adam Lehman, USA, talking about Applied Physiology

Applied Physiology (AP) is the work of one of Energy Kinesiology's earliest leading innovators, Richard Utt. With a strong integration between the neurological basis of kinesiology and the metaphysical energy model of the body/mind, Applied Physiology has contributed many ground breaking concepts to the field of Energy Kinesiology since its inception in the early 1980s. I want to tell you about just a couple of those innovations.

There are two main models in kinesiology: the indicator muscle model, where the practitioner uses a single muscle to communicate with the body globally, and the energy readout model, where each muscle expresses the energy flow in a specific, related meridian. AP marries these two models in a unique way that has now been adopted by other K systems. Initially, the indicator muscle is used to efficiently find imbalances, such as through the alarm points of Chinese medicine, and then the muscle related to the affected meridian is monitored to represent the actual neurological imbalance that was found using the indicator muscle. In this way, a more complete picture of the imbalance is established.

Another model that AP works with extensively is the holographic model (see page 31). While one could say that almost any of the healing arts work within the holographic model in some way, AP makes conscious use of this model by exploring, in a three dimensional structure, the relationships between the meridians affected by a person's issue.

By working in this three dimensional construct, the AP practitioner has the ability to accurately pinpoint where imbalances exist and then direct healing energy to those specific places, choosing from a variety of balancing techniques. As an example, if the practitioner were to find that the client's pectoralis major clavicular (PMC) has an imbalance, the practitioner would think of the stomach meridian due to its association with PMC. But the stomach meridian, with 45 meridian acupressure points, its relationship to the stomach organ, and several associated muscles, is a big picture with lots of possibilities! Applying balancing techniques to just 'the stomach' would be very generalised.

Using the holographic model, an AP practitioner identifies, using an indicator muscle, that the specific stomach imbalance is in relation to another meridian, e.g. the gall bladder. This immediately gives the practitioner a wealth of more information to consider relative to the imbalance – physiologically, emotionally or otherwise. As well - to further establish this relationship - Applied Physiology uses a 14 position range of motion for every muscle. Each position of a muscle relates that muscle's meridian to each of the other 14 meridians. As an example, to represent the neurological relationship of the stomach to the gall bladder, the PMC muscle would be placed in a specific position in its range of motion (position 4) and monitored there. In this way, an accurate representation of the imbalance in that relationship is achieved.

Another aspect of this three dimensional holographic model is similar to a hologram itself. If you cut up an actual exposed holographic plate into a hundred little pieces, each little piece still contains the whole, much like DNA. It will still present a full picture of the original object. However, as the pieces get smaller, the holographic picture gets fuzzier. In AP, each pair of meridians is like a piece of holographic film. By continuing to find information of different meridian relationships to an issue - it's like pulling together a lot of little pieces of holographic film to form a clearer picture of the whole. For the client, this means creating awareness about connections they may have never otherwise consciously established in relation to their issue. As a result, it's not unusual for a client to experience this as a series of 'Aha!s'. This effect may be encouraged with the assistance of verbal input from the practitioner, or simply happen because of the energy shifts that occur during the process itself.

A typical AP session uses the holographic model to identify where stressors exist, and then, using an indicator muscle as 'the voice of the subconscious', empowers the client to choose from a broad variety of balancing techniques, including physical, emotional and metaphysical, to provide a very thorough holistic balance. Tools common to an AP practitioner are tuning forks - specially developed by AP, emotional processing, energy systems such as the figure eights and the chakras (see page 08), and other healing modalities. Many of these are proprietary methods developed by Applied Physiology's originator, Richard Utt.

Additionally, one of the advantages of the holographic model is that it is an open system, and therefore allows easy integration of knowledge and techniques a practitioner may have learned in other healing or kinesiology modalities. As one of the early forms of Energy Kinesiology, Applied Physiology is a great gift to practitioners of the art of muscle monitoring.

Adam Lehman, Sonoma, California, USA
www.kinesiohealth.com/html/Programs/AP/aphome.html
www.kinesiohealth.com

Classical Kinesiology

Terry Larder, UK, talking about Classical Kinesiology

I've always been interested in all things medical and never wanted to work in an office environment but for various reasons ended up working in a hospital as a trainee hospital administrator. So I ended up in an office environment after all, and went on to work in the Highways Department of a local government - not what I would have considered exciting.

Looking back I realise that my interest in alternative medicine was rooted in my childhood. My mother used to buy Here's Health magazine before it became fashionable to be interested in naturopathy and introduced everyone who ate with us to yoghurt, using 'proper' yoghurt cultures that tasted tangy like sour grapes. I realise now what an influence my mother had been on me in those early years. With my deep rooted desire to help people, I was really excited when a friend came back from Canada thrilled with the new reflexology treatment and the health benefits she'd received. (This was 1980 and no one had heard of reflexology then). Knowing nothing at all about reflexology and with the support of my husband, I found out how to train and quickly found myself giving treatments in my living room - or anywhere there was a pair of feet! The results were amazing, and soon I was asking to go part-time at work so that I could expand my evening clinics to work 2 days a week.

After a few years as a reflexologist I realised that there were groups of people that I just couldn't help, and I felt that I needed more skills to be able to do so. I was also getting bored. In 1985 I learned about kinesiology when I was at an advanced reflexology seminar. Someone told me that there were reflex points on the body as well as the feet and that there was a kinesiology course going on in the next room. I decided I wanted to learn this new skill and promptly walked next door to ask for more information, only to find myself in the middle of a Touch for Health course.

I was absolutely fascinated by the courses. It took me a long time to get the hang of muscle testing, but all my reflexology patients were willing guinea-pigs. I was getting results that just took me to a whole new level of natural healthcare, and over the years I supplemented these courses with many others relating to the principles of naturopathy. I have never got tired of learning, because there is always something new to learn.

Despite giving many talks and teaching at the local community college from time to time, I always said I would never teach. However, with lots of pressure to provide kinesiology training outside of London, I conceded. In 1993 I started my own school, the Classical Kinesiology Institute (CKI), got the courses accredited by an awarding body and expanded the range of subjects to cover all that was required to become a competent practitioner. The kinesiology skills taught at the CKI are eclectic and cover the best in kinesiology research; we teach techniques that have stood the test of time as well as new ideas. Since then I have enjoyed seeing many students thrill at the 'magic' of kinesiology, make life changes, and make a good living as a kinesiology practitioner During this time period I was also chair of the Kinesiology Federation policy board and have given a total of 10 years' service over the past 25 years.

So I did achieve my childhood wish in the end, and I would not change anything. Kinesiology has been my life's work. Seeing thousands of patients achieve health improvements and experiencing the excitement of students could never ever have been surpassed by being trained in orthodox medicine.

Terry Larder, Leicestershire ,UK
www.classicalkinesiology.co.uk
www.turnaroundyourhealth.co.uk

Counselling Kinesiology

Counselling Kinesiology™, developed by Gordon and Debra Dickson, is a combination of mainstream and complementary counselling techniques, coaching and kinesiology. Gordon trained as an electrical engineer and worked as an orchestral musician in Australia and the Netherlands before he became involved with counselling and complementary therapies. Debra was originally a nurse before becoming a bodywork therapist and a homeopath.

Counselling Kinesiology™ uses muscle testing to test for emotional stress and to pinpoint the critical emotional references from the past that are causing the person to maintain the current problem emotions.

Counselling Kinesiology™ uses the Developmental Directory™ and Grief Gauge™ emotional states charts. These are used with muscle testing to identify the critical emotional states that have been internalised. The Developmental Directory™ is based on the psychosocial developmental stages. It identifies unmet emotional needs that prevented the development of emotional strengths and appropriate coping skills at particular phases of life. This lack of coping skills continues to cause problems throughout a person's life until they are addressed.

The Grief Gauge™ tracks the natural way a person comes to terms with any unwanted loss or change, including the specific tasks of grieving, to arrive at some type of narrative resolution. Muscle testing, using the Grief Gauge™, quickly identifies where this process has become stuck, and what is preventing the person satisfactorily coming to terms with the pain of the unwanted loss or change. The practitioner guides the clients through the grieving process, helping them connect with the emotional strengths they need to feel totally differently about the issue.

Although the focus is on the emotional and psychological, Counselling Kinesiology™ recognises that food and chemical sensitivities, learning issues, physical pain and ill-health can be associated with frustration and mood changes. It also recognises that emotional problems can underlie physical problems and that clearing emotional distress can lead to improvement in or elimination of physical symptoms.

Techniques include talk therapy, inner child work, use of flower remedies (see page 41), positive psychology and behaviour change exercises etc. Clients are taught practical skills that they can use in relationships, and to improve their own wellbeing and their ability to manage change and challenges.

www.counsellingkinesiology.com.au

Creative Kinesiology

Carrie Jost, UK, writing about Creative Kinesiology

In Creative Kinesiology we find an approach to healing and health that meets the individual with their story, their need to be witnessed in the traumas and life difficulties they have experienced and uses the techniques that suit their body, mind, spirit and feelings. How often have we not been heard, really listened to in a way that soothes and heals the soul? Creative Kinesiology attempts to do just that. Sessions focus entirely on the client's needs, and the approach is one of working together – client and practitioner co-creating the session by recognising what the client's body and mind are saying through the muscle testing approach used in all kinesiologies.

More than twenty years ago an acupuncturist called Haakon Lovell began to work in a new way. He had discovered muscle testing from an applied kinesiologist called Alan Beardall. He found that by getting this feedback from the energy systems of the people he was working with he could find clues from their sub-conscious and unconscious about what was happening to them. Since those early days we now have a real sense that the clues also come from the Higher Self, and are known by the parts of ourselves that are hidden from view. These are the parts that are accessible through muscle testing.

I worked with Haakon for several years in those early days of Creative Kinesiology and embarked on the same voyage of discovery about ways to work with people. The clues that emerged were compiled into a manual of files – called The Files. They are still used today and give us an amazing amount of information as we work with people. The companion manual is of Favourite Techniques that take us into the realms of the subtle energy (see page 08) of meridians and elements, the aura and chakras (see page 09 and 11 and 13 and 08). Added to this are ways of working with the nervous and endocrine systems, both of which act as intermediaries between the subtle energy systems and the physical body.

Our ancestors can be a source of gifting to us as well as a source of difficulty, and both the Files and the Favourite Techniques have information and techniques for this kind of work. One of the courses we follow in creative kinesiology is tracking to the origin of the problem, to the trigger that set the problem in motion. These make up the stories that may originate in childhood trauma, stresses and strains, accidents and all those other upsets that we encounter in life. Other trackways can take us back to our ancestral line, where the trigger amounts to trauma in our family line. These traumas can be very physical such as famine, injury or sheer hardship, or they can be emotional traumas such as loss and bereavement while spiritual trauma can include persecution or excommunication. The triggers are many and various. Solving the problems in the blood lineage is a very effective and economical way of healing - covering many generations in one go! Similar achievements for the 'spiritual lineage' can be deep and life changing as we find the roots of the healing needed for problems left over from past lives. Apart from the efficacy of this work, it is also interesting and revitalising for the person being helped.

Perceptual Bodywork (see page 74) is another aspect of the Creative Kinesiology approach and focuses on a sensing approach to the more physical aspects of problems. It builds on the Applied Kinesiology material and protocols.

As we discover the story behind a person's symptoms, whether it be illness, depression, aches and pains, low energy, stress, migraines or inability to make relationships, we edge our way to the trigger point that caused the problem to arise. The journey is one made by the client and the practitioner together, co-creating the way forward, finding the clues and witnessing whatever is present for the person. The fact that the Creative Kinesiology sessions are part of a journey means that we, with our clients, work towards resolution, health and happiness over a period of time. The work is a process of discovery, renewal and inspiration.

Central to the work of Creative Kinesiology is the concept of life journey – and recognises that we are all on a path. Finding the path that is right for us seems to be the work of the moment. Many people are seeking, and this is one of the ways in which the seeker may be helped to find what they are looking for. In Creative Kinesiology we use maps that are recognised by the person's system. This helps with the tracking process, so we can follow the pathways to any blockages and stoppages in the system. One of the maps takes us to the relevant tracking level we need to investigate, whether it be the body's systems, the biochemical makeup of the cells or the spiritual level of finding meaning and purpose in life. Another map allows us to discover the environmental influences that are affecting us such as geopathic stress (see page 35), ley lines or the type of water we are drinking. Once we have found the blockage and the nature of the problem we can use energy techniques to heal and transform so the system can flow along its rightful path.

The Creative Kinesiologist is a tracker, standing alongside the person, travelling the terrain of the individual's story with them, looking for the clues that tell us why the person is not on their track. We know we are on track when we are feeling good about life. With the clues and the techniques available it is possible to help the person rediscover their purpose, their dream to aim for and to restore their sense of meaning in life.

Creative Kinesiology has been taught to students as a professional training course for twenty years. Those embarking on the training are those who are willing to go through their own journey of discovery and inner growth. We now have a Foundation course for those who wish to do this for themselves, or as a prelude to professional training. We have called this series of workshops Lifetracking. It is open to anyone interested in their own journey and possibly sharing the approaches and techniques with family and friends or as a first step to becoming a professional kinesiologist.

Within Creative Kinesiology we run two professional training courses. One called Way of the Tracker using the approach of working with the Files as clues to the person's condition – the other Perceptual Bodywork takes a more physical approach. Together they provide a thorough training in kinesiology, offering a personally designed healing, designed on the spot, as the practitioner follows the clues and discovers the way that healing will work for each individual.

Carrie Jost, Devon, UK
www.creativekinesiology.org

Creative Kinesiology: Judith Hart, UK, Case Study

Betty (not her real name) presented with strong anxiety, restlessness and neck pain, saying that her life was in a mess and she didn't know which way to turn. Betty is self-employed and was worried about money and the direction in which to take her business, as she works in a couple of different areas of the country. The situation was becoming intolerable, as she was getting tired out with the travelling. She knew she needed to drop one area of her work. However, she felt split; she didn't know how to divide her time and was worried that releasing herself from the travelling would result in a drop in her income. She couldn't seem to get organized enough to sort anything out or make any real choices; she felt she just couldn't make any decisions.

On starting the session we immediately found that her spleen meridian was out of balance, and that this was affecting her faith in the future. The meridian had become over-energised, so that she was experiencing surges of anxious energy. We also found that her gall bladder meridian was out of balance. The gall bladder meridian governs decision-making, choice and step by step planning in life, so the fact that this meridian was not working properly in that area made sense to the client. By using the tool of muscle-testing we found that other emotions that were unbalancing her were feelings of impotency and helplessness. These emotions are associated with the gall bladder meridian, and Betty said that was just how she was feeling.

We then found some fear had surfaced around her realizing her dreams and achieving her potential in life. She hopes to go on to be a writer and is in the process of writing something, which she wishes to get published. It turned out that some weeks ago she had made the decision to stop travelling so much with her business so that she could concentrate more on her writing and building her business in one place. At the time she had been happy about this decision, and it was a feasible move financially, but she had suddenly exploded into worry about it all.

Further investigation through muscle-testing revealed that she was experiencing an internal split and therefore was unable to carry through her initial plan of following her dream. All the different parts of herself were not aligned with what she wanted to do, allowing fear to rule the show. She was essentially divided, rather than united behind what she wanted. The muscle-testing also showed us that this was an unconscious archetypal pattern held deep within her system, the type of pattern which humans feel as a need to divide and fragment, rather than unite and co-create.

On realizing that she had gone into an unconscious pattern, she gave a huge sigh of relief and visibly came to life again and started to smile, after having been very pale when she entered the session. She said that she suddenly felt whole again and much lighter and relieved. Her gall bladder and spleen meridians were balanced using techniques from the Touch for Health system and further muscle-testing showed that the emotions of helplessness and impotency that were knocking her off centre had come back into balance. Betty confirmed this by saying that she felt totally different, and that her shoulders and back had loosened up and she had more flexibility to turn her neck.

Betty has since made good progress with her writing and has completed her first draft. She is now considering looking for a publisher. She has not experienced a return to the worried state she was in when she came for the session; she has organised a number of work projects for the future in the area where she lives. Being happy with her decision to reduce the travelling she was doing, Betty has also been able to consolidate her work closer to home and is more relaxed and happier for it. She is supporting herself at home with some energy exercises I showed her. These strengthen the meridians and help keep the mind clear. She is also continuing to have maintenance treatments every couple of months to make sure she stays on track.

Judith Hart, Devon, UK
www.mayanastrology.co.uk

Ali Ashby, UK, talking about Creative Kinesiology

I'd had my daughter allergy tested by a kinesiologist in Sussex when we lived there. When we moved to Exeter I wanted her re-tested, so I took Evie, who was then 18 months old, to see Carrie Jost. It was my first experience of Creative Kinesiology, and I was blown away by the way she worked. Carrie tracked through Evie's system to find out what was going on at a wider level, not just with allergies. This was 9 years ago, and in that moment I knew I wanted to train in this amazing way of working.

At the time I was working as a psychosynthesis therapeutic counsellor and so was used to working in depth helping people explore their soul's journey. I felt I could bring the two together.

I signed up to train with Carrie and did the Touch for Health courses first, as was a requirement at the time. Now the Creative Kinesiology School offers a course called Life Tracking, which replaces the TFH courses for people who know they want to train in Creative Kinesiology, as well as offering a way into kinesiology and working with subtle energy for people wanting to work on their own personal journey. (I helped develop that with Carrie Jost and Judith Hart.)

I like Creative Kinesiology because it is out of the box, and not protocol based. When you're the practitioner, you don't know where you're going – you're following the client's inner wisdom and journey, working in a co-creative way and very much 'in the moment'. It means weaving between different realms, so, for example, we might start working in the physical realm, move to the emotional and then electromagnetic, before moving back to the emotional – and so on. In this way, we 'tell the story' of the particular issue that the client would like to explore, and it can be an eye-opener for people to acknowledge that there is a complex story behind the 'symptom' that has brought them to the session. It is in the witnessing of this story that greater understanding and healing is possible.

I worked as a Creative Kinesiology practitioner for six years, and then I started teaching Life Tracking. I'd never seen myself as a teacher, but Creative Kinesiology opened this up for me and made me want to share this work with people in a group setting.

I liked the training because it was non-linear - going with whatever was upper-most for the group, so the learning felt very experiential and relevant in the 'here and now'. I felt I absorbed it on a body as well as a head level. Now that I've started teaching Way of the Tracker, I am loving this way of working from the 'teacher' end as much as I did from the 'student' end!

The Touch for Health and Creative Kinesiology courses were spread out over about 18 months, which made it relatively easy to combine the training with being a mum and working part time as a therapist. I changed a lot over that time – coming to know more of my self - as the CK course is very much a journey of self-discovery as well as learning how to be a professional kinesiologist. I had done a lot of work on myself in my psych synthesis training, and the CK training deepened my journey further through the experience of witnessing the various 'stories' that I explored during this time, both on a personal and group level.

I have clients from three years of age to 84, and I really like that - the whole age range. I also love the fact that it empowers people to understand their own journey more, to become co-creative. It's not about doing something to someone and the client doesn't understand what you are doing, and people often take away tools they can use, so they can really be part of it.

It feels a huge privilege to me to be able to accompany people in the process of understanding more about themselves and what they need to do to come into balance. I like the fact that people come with such a huge range of 'issues': from pain, to stress, to insomnia, to feeling 'stuck in life', and the training teaches you to use tracking skills to explore whatever the client brings.

Ali Ashby, Devon, UK

Rachel Lead, UK, writing about Creative Kinesiology/Perceptual Bodywork

Perceptual Bodywork was created by Natalie Davenport using the skills acquired through her many years of training in bodywork. The techniques are based on advanced Touch for Health and a simplified form of Applied Kinesiology. This bodywork is a separate division to Way of The Tracker and links to The School of Creative Kinesiology. The main aim is to follow the person's health history through muscle testing. The road to fuller health and recovery is a two way partnership between the practitioner and person, hence this case study is written in the plural. The use of perception through the senses, muscle testing and corrections enables the clearance of old issues and injuries. This promotes natural healing and personal development for the client.

Mark (not his real name) is over 50 years old. He described his main issues and problems as being depression, panic attacks, bi-polar symptoms (which he explained as slightly manic for several days, followed by days in depression), food sensitivity, feelings of unworthiness and feeling ugly, feeling switched off, inactive, as though something was in his way. He was also lacking in confidence, and looking around all the time as though being watched or followed.

Mark is interested in history and researching his family tree, so he was particularly drawn to our work of re-patterning and changing his perception of his life story. He always turns up for his appointment with a list of areas connected to family issues past and present that he wants us to explore. When he first started coming to see me the wording was 'family tree'. Over a period of time he developed this into 'family tree and ancestors', and now Mark asks that all corrections used are not only for himself, but for his family tree, ancestors and all distantly related ancestors and relatives.

I have seen this client regularly over several years and the session below is a typical example of the areas we have worked on.

We start a session by talking about the subject of the moment (the goal). The posture is then observed, and that day there was an uneven torque or twisting within the body. Mark described his energy as: "frenetic, like metal balls bouncing around and off the body".

During a session, either I or the client may arrive at something by reasoning or by using our intuition, or we may use the Perceptual Bodywork map, but the next action is always decided through muscle testing. Even if a client says: 'Oh I know what that is I have been to another therapist and they said...' the next step or correction is always confirmed with muscle testing.

Our starting point in Perceptual Bodywork was in the personal ecology realm, and we used corrections for the adrenal syndrome mode (to help reduce stress and exhaustion in the body). I asked if he was aware of any tension in his body. He said that he was aware of tension in his head and jaw area (common areas when stress is involved). The use of therapy locating on his body confirmed this. The related kidney and adrenals area switched off the indicator muscle. I tested muscles related to the triple warmer meridian, because these are usually out of balance in adrenal stress. Any unlocked muscles were corrected first. Then the adrenal exhaustion points (AEP) were held. While the various AEP points were being held, Mark's body had convulsions of energy, until eventually the internal forces equalised. On re-testing, the previously switched off areas held against an indicator muscle. Mark said that he 'felt free to fight', as he had previously revealed that he was late in speaking, very quiet and passive, allowing others to complete tasks for him. The words 'free to fight' imply that he has broken free of this pattern of acceptance, as the stress of the imprint from his family history had been released.

Next Mark had a memory taking him back to the age of 3 years - he was not happy, was forlorn and low in energy. The technique needed was in the emotional realm (ER) and heart appreciation was used. This involves the person thinking of a positive memory, and we really had to search to find one! The appropriate memory was confirmed through muscle testing.

After completing the heart appreciation correction, the ER finger mode (see page 21) was still not holding against an indicator muscle test – it was switching off. Muscle testing indicated that Mark did not need another correction from the emotional realm file or more of the heart appreciation. Using finger modes for the different realms the indicator muscle switched off for the next priority, the electromagnetic realm (EL-R). When we muscle tested through the various techniques in the EL-R, the indicator muscle showed that we needed to work with the technique 'working in & off the body'.

This is to facilitate detailed corrections on the body that are not possible to touch directly. An anatomy book is often used to help with visualisation, unless the kinesiologist knows the physiology of the body well. By tuning into the aura (see page 13) and the subtle vibration of the body parts, we can establish the place for healing, which was confirmed by muscle testing. This was the top left chamber of the heart, which Mark said felt squidgy, and the appropriate technique of two pointing was used. This involves connecting two parts of the body to jump-start natural healing. Mark held the heart area, and I held the Emotional Stress Release points on the forehead. Whilst holding these points, we talked a lot to find the right word – suppression. When this was said by him, tiny convulsions in all the muscles of the body seemed to occur, freeing up bodily movements.

 In any Perceptual Bodywork session it is important for the practitioner to know when to talk and when to be silent, so that clients have the time to work out for themselves the best way forward. You can help by muscle testing to find the appropriate area of discussion, but I always wait, sometimes for ages, for the client to find and say the word or words.

After using these corrections the ER and the EL-R finger modes were checked by muscle testing and were now holding.

After that Mark walked around the room and looked at his posture and became aware of new flexibility and release of tension in some areas of his body. The session was coming to a close. We checked the goal and all the related issues that had been talked about in the session. Through the use of muscle testing we confirmed that all was well with him before he left.

Mark has described the PB process as like a stone mason chiselling, and slowly there you are, revealed as your true self.

Now that we have worked together for some time, Mark describes his original issues and problems like this:

> "Depression - 100% cleared.
> "Panic attacks - 100% cleared.
> "Bi-polar symptoms (ie slightly manic for several days, followed by days in depression) - 85% cleared.
> "Food sensitivity - 90% cleared - no longer an issue for me.
> "Feelings of unworthiness/feeling ugly - 100% cleared.
> "Feeling switched off/inactive, as though something was in my way - 95% cleared.

"I would say these were my most important symptoms. They were reduced by percentage points as we tackled different issues. Negative changes were re-experiencing the symptoms briefly as we tackled them. It was like having a time machine. They only ever lasted a few days though.
 "As for what's left to change - not a lot!"

Rachel Lead, Oxfordshire, UK
www.chilterntherapy.co.uk

Crossinology® - Brain Integration Technique

Crossinology's Brain Integration Technique (BIT) was developed by Susan J. McCrossin. After collaborating with Dr Charles Krebs (see page 50) she developed her own system and moved to the USA.

BIT uses muscle testing, acupressure points and mudras to diagnose and correct learning difficulties, including ADD, ADHD and Dyslexia. It is based on a neurological understanding of the how the brain is not working as it should and uses the meridian system to correct the dysfunction. The model is supported by research with brain scanning showing abnormal brain activity whilst performing a cognitive task prior to treatment and normal brain activity post treatment. Having had a learning difficulty herself, Susan has a particular insight into what it is like living with a learning difficulty, and the lack of function that results.

BIT takes between 8 and 12 hours, depending on the individual. It can be done all at once (over two or three days), or spread out over a longer period of time.

www.crossinology.com

Susan J. McCrossin talking about working with two clients:

Carol M.'s ten-year-old son, Alex, had been diagnosed with ADHD and put on Ritalin at age nine. She brought him to me from their home in California for a weekend of intensive therapy. After ten hours of treatment, she stopped giving him Ritalin 'cold turkey'. No one ever suspected her son wasn't using the medication anymore because his behavior was normal, and he went from making C's and D's in school to earning B's. The treatment changed her son's life. As Carol says: "The liberation from a lifelong label is a priceless gift. It allows the child to create a life that is driven by their passion and not their arbitrary diagnosis."

When I met Lauren in April 2003, she was fifteen years old. A competitive figure skater, she was quite sociable and had many friends at school, but she had suffered from very poor reading comprehension and difficulty expressing herself verbally throughout her school years. Test and performance anxiety were big problems, too. She had trouble with math, especially memorizing her times tables, and she scored at a fourth-grade equivalency for mathematics reasoning and numerical operations on a WISC IIIR assessment. The assessment placed her vocabulary at the fifth percentile and her comprehension at the thirty-seventh percentile, roughly at a third- or fourth-grade level. Her processing speed scores, however, were quite good, placing her at the ninety-seventh percentile, and she had good auditory memory. A psychologist who tested Lauren described her as having "a mild language disorder which … encompasses problems with expressing word meanings and concept formations as well as the misapplication of grammatical rules and syntax and relatively poor language comprehension." Upon initial assessment, I found Lauren needed correction to sort out the confusion about which side of her brain performed logic functions and which side performed creative, or

Gestalt, functions; the messages being sent were all crossed. She had very low (4 per cent) access to pathways in the corpus callosum. Her Gestalt hemisphere, testing at 100 per cent access, was dominant over her logic hemisphere, which could access just 64 per cent overall. She had only 7 per cent access to pathways dealing with reading comprehension and 8 per cent access to arithmetic functions. After treatment, these pathways were restored to 100 per cent access.

Lauren's case illustrates the impact that brain integration has on overall well-being. When Lauren returned home, one of the first things she did was take a driving test for her learner's permit. She read the rules-of-the-road book without any help and passed the test with only three mistakes. She was especially pleased because a number of the items on the test were multiple-choice questions, a format she had struggled with previously. About a month after treatment, her mom wrote to me, "Lauren is starting to see for herself some of the wonderful positive effects of our visit to you. Her math tutor says she is far more focused and much more readily grasps concepts that before were difficult. Lauren herself says it is a real treat to read her history text – once- and understand what she reads - and remember what she read!! She feels very happy … in control … and not in angst at all about final exams which start this week." This from a girl who previously suffered significant test anxiety!

Susan J McCrossin, Boulder, Colorado, USA
Author of *Breaking the Learning Barrier: Eradicating ADD, ADHD and Dyslexia*
www.crossinology.com

Cyberkinetics

Dr Diego Vellam, Italy, writing about Cyberkinetics

My name is Diego Vellam. I am the director and founder of the Academy of Kinesiology in Italy, and the president and founder of the Federation of Kinesiology, a non-profit organization recognized by the Italian government. I have also been serving for years on the board of directors of the International Association of Specialized Kinesiologists (I-ASK). My initial studies have been in physics, though. I got my PhD in solid state physics, specializing in surface (molecular) physics, with a keen interest in the quantum mechanics aspects of reality. Physics has always been for me an important tool in approaching reality.

I distinctly recall my first class in kinesiology. Actually I didn't even mean to get there, it was my bride (just married) that asked me to join her in "this new thing", and so I did. The course was embarrassingly lousy, just like the instructor. Yet, being accustomed to "weird" theories in physics, I knew that the only way to judge validity is to give it a try. When so doing, this new stuff worked, and well. So I got hooked, and spent the next years taking kinesiology classes around the world, pursuing my own personal research.

This led me to founding the Academy of Kinesiology in Milano, Italy, and for its classes I have developed so far more than twenty new kinesiology courses that have been successfully taught to lots of students through the years.

It was in 2000 that I got to know what, in my personal experience, I regard as the most advanced kinesiology system that has been developed so far. At a conference someone talked about new ways of testing that had been just developed within a new kinesiology called Cyberkinetics. The moment I tried this new Analogue Test (see page 15) I couldn't but realize that a real quantum leap had just taken place in kinesiology.

As I got to know the name Cyberkinetics derives from cybernetics and kinesiology; its purpose is to address the multi-level cybernetic processes that take place in the human being with new ways of kinesiology testing, expressly developed for this purpose. Since cybernetics represents the science of communication and control processes within systems, it explicitly deals with the factors behind homeostasis and hence health. The final result is a new kinesiology system that is at the same time simple, efficient and effective.

I immediately got in contact with the person who had been developing that, an Englishman named Alan Sales. That was the start of a deep mutual collaboration that kept us investigating on the frontiers of kinesiology for the next nine years, until his untimely death on July 7th, 2009.

Right away I started teaching the first available course, Cyberkinetics – Module 1, to audiences of kinesiologists in awe of the strikingly effective and simple, though revolutionary, approach. Year after year other modules followed, each one of them literally pushing further the limits of what had been considered possible in kinesiology. The seventh and final module, Cyberkinetics – The 7th Wave, has been developed by me on the basis of original and still unpublished research work of Alan Sales. This module was taught for the first time in 2010, one year after Alan's unexpected departure. It introduces the Concurrency Test, which represents the peak of all the communication tools that have been developed within Cyberkinetics.

Every one of the Cyberkinetics modules offers amazing insights into the resources available to each human being, showing how to tap into them effectively in order to facilitate the healing process. Analogue Test, Cyberkinetic Test, Molecular Test and Concurrency Test have all been conceived to the benefit of all kinesiologists, and can be independently employed as such also in different kinesiology systems. The results that can be achieved quickly and easily using these unique Cyberkinetics tests are just amazing.

Alan Sales did not limit his seminal contributions to kinesiology only. For all his life he had been very interested in the healing power of sound, and so he designed an amazing system of special tuning forks that have been produced by a nearby manufacturer with four centuries of experience in harmonic alloy. To this purpose he crafted no less than 321 special tuning forks grouped in 25 different sets, with matching healing protocols that represent the top in sound therapy.

With all due blessings to the dear memory of Alan Sales, one of the greatest innovators in kinesiology.

Dr Diego Vellam, Milano, Italy
www.cyberkinetics.it
www.diapasonterapia.it
www.accademiadikinesiologia.it
www.federazionedikinesiologia.org

Dynamic Healing

Barbara Grimwade, Spain, writing about Dynamic Healing

Wow, Kinesiology really works! That was my 'Road to Damascus' moment. Having been a scientist for many years, I never believed in alternative therapies and even less expected them to be effective.

I suffered with minor health problems for years, an occasional bad back, frequent headaches and recurrent thrush. I didn't want to make a fuss over what I saw as minor things, so I just put up with them, took a few painkillers and carried on as normal. I didn't realise then that it was my body's way of telling me that something wasn't right with my life.

Over time my symptoms got much worse and I ended up being off work for months with back strain, although it wasn't until I developed full-blown Candida (which gave me a whole myriad of nasty symptoms) that I turned to the medical profession. The doctor pumped me so full of drugs that I could have opened a pharmacy. And what did they do for me? Absolutely nothing! In fact, my symptoms got a lot worse. I was in a terrible state and, after one back manipulation, I was told that I might never walk properly again, and I didn't for a long time.

On top of this I was feeling lousy. I had developed migraines, felt bloated and not in control of my life anymore. At the time I was a research scientist in molecular biology, and had been for many years. I had been very intuitive as a young woman, but that was bred out of me when I started studying science, as I was taught to be logical and analytical about everything. I followed this train of thought for many years and, even though I was passionate about biology, I became increasingly disillusioned with my work.

We were at the beginning of the genetic modification phase and, although my colleagues were enthusiastic about it, I had my doubts way back before GM ever hit the headlines. As I didn't really know what else to do, I carried on with my job for a few more years and it was during this time that my health deteriorated further.

As you can imagine, as a scientist I was initially utterly sceptical about non-conventional therapies. However, a homeopath friend convinced me to at least try a different route. So, very reluctantly, I began to investigate complementary and alternative therapies, though more through desperation than anything else. This investigation was to last five years, as I tried virtually every therapy that there was. Some helped a little, some didn't, but I was now firmly on that path, searching for relief.

Throughout my search, I kept hearing about kinesiology. "Kinesy-what?" I thought. It sounded a bit too strange to me. You put your arm out and someone can tell what's going on by the response? I don't think so! So I kept on searching, and kinesiology kept on cropping up. I read that it was one of the only therapies that was effective for Candida, but still I wouldn't try it. However, one day, five years into my search, I was at a workshop where the organiser told me that she had found a kinesiologist locally and that the treatment had made a huge difference to her health. That was my cue to finally try this strange sounding therapy.

Right from the beginning of the treatment I had a sense that I was in the right place, as the kinesiologist guided me through an amazing process. She touched on parts of my psyche that I hardly recognised, although deep down I knew that it all resonated with a truth I had known for ever, but had somehow forgotten.

In a couple of sessions, we had identified nutritional deficiencies and some work-related stress that were contributing to my physical symptoms. However, more importantly, we had cleared years of emotional baggage, which was the main cause; and I had thought I had my emotional life pretty sorted up until then!

I found it absolutely amazing. I'd identified, and dealt with, the reason I kept getting into the same situation again and again, a self-sabotage that was easily treated. It was as if a weight that I hadn't even known I'd been carrying had been lifted and I felt fantastic. My symptoms disappeared completely and, in 15 years, have never come back.

Kinesiology rapidly addressed the underlying reasons that were causing my symptoms – a lack of fulfilment in my work, and a lack of direction as to where I wanted to be. After eight years of suffering, within two sessions my symptoms had almost gone. My reaction was definite, this stuff worked! I was so impressed at the change it made, not only to my physical health but also to my emotional and spiritual well-being that I wanted to learn it so I could help others.

I signed up for a course in Classical Kinesiology the following week and have never looked back! The training itself was exhilarating and I couldn't get enough of it. I couldn't wait for the next module. Everything seemed to make so much sense, and having knowledge of human physiology made it easy to link everything together. Coming from a scientific background, I understood the concept of energy, at least at a molecular level, and the idea that everything is connected was never a problem for me.

After studying Kinesiology, nutrition and counselling skills I became a practitioner in my own right. I then went on to qualify in several different advanced kinesiologies, Emotional Freedom Technique, and Neuro-Linguistic programming amongst others. I moulded the best of these philosophies together with my experience; into a system I call Dynamic Healing. I now practise this on Mallorca. Looking back, it was the best decision I ever made. I love my life and my 'work' is my passion. I can never imagine doing anything else.

Barbara Grimwade, Calvia, Mallorca, Spain
www.dynamic-healing.com

Health Kinesiology

Health Kinesiology was developed by Jimmy Scott, Ph.D., a physiological psychologist from the USA.

HK practitioners make extensive use of verbal questioning (see page 22), possibly to a greater extent than any other kinesiology practitioners. The use of finger modes (see page 21) is not taught in HK. Unlike many kinesiologists, HK practitioners usually work with over energy rather than under energy. First the meridian energy system is balanced, and then practitioners use muscle testing with verbal questioning to establish permission from the energy system to proceed and the best way to proceed. They may work on the client's presenting problem or use verbal questioning to establish what the priority is for the energy system.

HK has its own specific pre-tests. Once the initial pre-tests are completed, the session can be organised in various ways. The session can be organized by simple priority – muscle testing and verbal questioning are used to establish the priority thing to do (usually an energy correction), then the next and the next, until there is nothing more to do then or the time runs out. The second way is working according to an issue decided by the client – this is often a presenting symptom or illness. The third way is to work according to issue priority established by the body through muscle testing. The fourth way is to work using causal analysis, which breaks down all the factors relevant to the client's presenting problem and analyses what needs to be done for each of them.

The HK practitioner uses a flow chart 'menu' to establish what type of work is needed. The possibilities are divided into four distinct categories or factors: energy corrections, energy toning, adjunctives and energy redirection. Within each category there is a further menu of techniques and procedures which are offered to the body for it to select through muscle testing.

Bio-energetic corrections are procedures which are done by the practitioner and/or with the client. Energy corrections form by far the most important category in terms of treatment. Each time the practitioner identifies a stress through muscle testing, triggers it in a controlled manner and then removes the stress permanently. During corrections clients may have to think something, place their hands on their bodies in a particular manner or have something placed on them - magnets, homeopathic remedies and crystals are just some of the possibilities. While this is happening the practitioner (and sometimes the client) will hold or tap specific places on the body. Sometimes Cosmic Batteries are used instead. Cosmic Batteries are subtle energy devices made in Belgium. Each Cosmic Battery (or Cos Bat, as they are called by HK practitioners) is a glass tube containing coloured coils, homeopathic remedies, coloured sand, symbols, etc. The HK practitioner tests for the correct one or ones to put on, or occasionally just off, the body. These have the effect of helping the system to regain balance.

Bio-energetic toning factors are things which the person goes away and does to tone their energy system. Aerobic exercise tones the physical body; energy toning tones the other subtle bodies (see page 08). As with physical exercise they may need to be done repeatedly to strengthen the energy of these bodies.

Adjunctive factors are also things which the clients do for themselves. Whereas energy toning exercises can affect the physical body through an indirect route, adjunctive factors affect the physical body directly. Physical exercise, nutrition, herbal supplements all primarily affect the physical body and so are classified as adjunctives. The practitioner uses muscle testing to determine which dietary change, supplement or exercise, etc. the person needs. Many HK practitioners also consider bio-energetic environmental factors, such as geopathic stress (see page 35) and psychic protection (where the client may need to be protected from the disturbing effect of other people or energies).

Bio-energetic redirection procedures are used where the energy of the body is directed to some specific goal which may not be of the highest priority for the body. This is only undertaken after the body has given specific permission to do so.

The HK practitioner always checks for energy permission to end a session and will continue working if this is not given.

www.HK-Training.org
www.HK-Practitioners.net
www.hk4health.co.uk

Dr Jimmy Scott, Canada, talking about Health Kinesiology

I have a PhD in Physiological Psychology and worked as a scientist for a number of years in medical–school type settings. I saw kinesiology demonstrated and was fascinated but skeptical and couldn't see how it could be used practically even if it did work.

Early 1977 I organized a demonstration by Chris Harrison, a Californian Applied Kinesiology Chiropractor. He made it very clear how it could be used, and I knew I had to learn how to do that to determine for myself if it worked. Chris suggested some material to read and to take a class. I did that, and it did seem to work. At that time I was also working as a nutritional consultant, using hair analysis to establish my clients' mineral balance. I decided to try muscle testing to find this information. I got the same answers as the lab tests, so that convinced me that it worked.

I realized that kinesiology does work if certain things are done properly, but nobody was sure what those certain things were! That was in 1977. In early 1978 I discovered how to do verbal questioning (see page 22) and that allowed me to progress much faster. I wanted to do certain things that no one seemed to know how to do. I used indices in my scientific work to compare different things, so I did the same in kinesiology, since with verbal questioning I could.

I was still working with nutrition and came across nutritional reflex points, which allow you to establish a client's need for particular supplements, e.g. calcium. I used this technique, but found that sometimes clients came back and were even worse. I realised that the form of the calcium didn't matter for the test, but did matter for the client. I realized I needed more precision. With muscle testing and verbal questioning I could be vastly more precise, establishing exactly which brand, dose, time of day …. Results were far better. I was excited!

Nutrition is not everything about a person's life. If nutrition is not what is needed, then what is? I took a scientific approach – what factors are important for a person? If indexing shows that nutrition is 5%, what is the rest? It may be psychological, infections, toxicity, exercise, rest, geobiology, which I brought into kinesiology about 1985 (see page 35) … I delineated each of these factors, and others. Verbal questioning helped me analyze what was going on for the client. I learned a lot about how to ask questions, but at first it was like a pioneer hacking a path slowly through a jungle - everything was a jumble, but gradually things became clearer and more effective.

In 1978 I developed a phobia correction that was based on my previous scientific experience – it combined psychological procedures (relaxation and systematic desensitization) with energy concepts. The results were even better than I expected, so that gave me even more confidence about what I was doing. That same scientific knowledge underlies virtually all of HK.

In 1980 I developed a way of detecting and correcting allergies. A woman came to see me who was allergic to almonds – eating them resulted in a pain in her shoulder. I thought about how we did psychological corrections, made an analogy and came up with the Symbiotic Energy Transformation™ procedure (SET). The procedure went well. In fact I was really surprised at how successful it was. In the early 1980's homeopathic versions of foods became available. I realized I could use these rather than actual substances. I still really hadn't appreciated how powerful the SET procedure was. A client came in and I said: "Let's fix all your allergies today." She agreed, and we did an SET with perhaps 200 things. The next day she phoned me, from the hospital; the medics had said she was haemorrhaging internally. A scan had shown she had a large endometrioma, and the medics wanted to operate. I felt she was experiencing a healing reaction and encouraged her to wait. The next day the severe pain had gone away and her blood tests were normal. She was discharged. Two weeks later she went to see her gynaecologist. He couldn't find the endometrioma. It had completely gone.

I carried on my research and began to realise how important priority and energy permission were. In 1984 I established the basic template for all energy corrections. We energy balance, find and then stimulate the stress (see page 32) and concurrently apply the energy correction. I also differentiated between energy corrections and energy toning. My quantum physics based theoretical model of the energy system was first published in 1984, and has been developed extensively since then.

I've carried on developing new corrections and ways of working with the person and analyzing what is happening and what is needed. Most of HK has been developed because of a need of a client – I use my knowledge from my scientific background and my imagination and use energy concepts with dramatically effective results. I've always read a lot and had a lot of different interests, so that has helped me find new procedures, new ways of doing things. I've incorporated so much of my own personal interests into HK and that's why it's been so much fun and so rewarding for all these years. Seeing clients change has been deeply rewarding.

Dr Jimmy Scott, Ontario, Canada
www.hk-training.org
www.HK-Practitioners.net

Ann Parker, New Zealand, talking about Health Kinesiology

Initially I wasn't looking for training in any natural therapy. I trained as a mathematician but had moved on to owning a very busy gift shop. I had developed very painful tennis elbows, and people kept telling me I should do something different. I saw an HK practitioner about my elbows, but she didn't get permission to work on them. She also told me that I needed a change of direction and suggested I train as a health kinesiologist. I thought "I could do this", even though I knew nothing about nutrition or anatomy and physiology. It really appealed to me because the practitioner works sitting down. My back was broken when I was 21, and I wouldn't have been able to work standing up and lifting people's legs into position, particularly if they were on the large side. I also liked the fact that the body itself guides you where you need to go, where you need to work in that person's best interest. So, I booked for my first HK course.

The night I posted the cheque off was the first night for months that I had not woken up weeping with the pain, and from then until the class they just got better and better.

On the first day of the course I thought: "This is something special. I could do this." By the end of the second day I thought: "If I get my act together, I could teach this." Teaching has been a life-long passion of mine; I taught in the main-stream educational system for 12 years before becoming a shop keeper. In fact I was becoming bored with the shop and had been thinking of going back to university and updating my skills so I could teach mathematics again. I was hooked right from that first HK course and wanted to teach that instead of maths.

A month after doing the first course, I did two courses with Dr Scott who was over from Canada. Then I worked really hard to get the hours and experience so that I could become a teacher. I saw lots of clients, attended all the HK courses, studied anatomy and physiology and nutrition, and sat in with some of the more experienced practitioners while they worked. My focus completely changed from being a shop keeper to being a health kinesiologist.

Once I started teaching I could see that the students became as excited as I was about HK. I saw how they changed as they worked on themselves. All that gave me great satisfaction and reinforced my belief that I was doing the right thing.

Over the next few years I started to employ more staff in the shop so that I could see more clients and be free to teach at weekends. I've been teaching HK since January 1994 and still feel passionate and excited about what HK can do, not just for clients but also for students – people change and grow as they work on themselves; their whole lives change for the better.

I used to see a lot of clients every day. I might have several with the same symptoms, but using the HK menu I'd do different things. The way the person got to that point is unique to them, so they have their own unique healing path to follow too. I could never have decided that with a head decision. This is one of the things that still amazes me about HK. Today, for example, I had a client who had to sniff an essential oil. When I read out the profile for that oil, it was her emotional profile exactly. The client said: "That's scary." I never get bored; the client's energy system always chooses the right thing.

I've made many really good friendships through HK. For the last seven years that I lived in the UK I was head of HK in the UK and also ran the Open College Network programme. I've now relocated to New Zealand and am looking forward to introducing people here and in Australia to the joy and wonders of HK.

Ann Parker, Wanaka, New Zealand
www.healthkinesiology.co.nz

Health Kinesiology: Vera Peiffer, UK, Case Study

Mrs M.H. (47) came to see me for Health Kinesiology. She had been having problems with her hair since giving birth to her third child, and over the last five years she had lost a lot of hair. Conventional therapy with Minoxidil made even more hair fall out, and iron supplementation prescribed by a hair specialist only resulted in limited improvement of her diffuse hair loss. When I checked her, it turned out that she had two amalgams and one gold filling and that she suffered from mercury toxicity. I explained to her that amalgam and gold is a particularly bad combination as the different metals create electric currents in the mouth that disturb the body's functioning. My client had the amalgam fillings changed for white fillings, and we tested for the right detoxifying herbs for her to take for six weeks after the dental treatment. We also worked with Health Kinesiology to help the body detoxify more efficiently and to re-balance her electro-magnetic field which had been disturbed by the metals in her mouth.

After four Health Kinesiology sessions, her hair was visibly darker and fuller. She did not have to take iron supplements any more as the Health Kinesiology helped her body to metabolise iron correctly from the food she eats.

A few weeks after her last Health Kinesiology session, she wrote to me.

"Dear Vera,
I want to thank you for the amazing change in my hair after only 4 sessions of treatment.
As you know I have had diffuse hair loss for many years and sought the help of a trichologist over a 4 year period. Despite following a programme of treatment with the trichologist including expensive hair drops and iron supplements, improvement in my hair over this period was disappointing and short lived.

I cannot pretend to entirely understand health kinesiology, but I can understand the outcome. I am fortunate to have an enormous amount of new hair growth and significantly, the quality of the new hair is the best I have had in years. The icing on the cake is that the hair coming through is my old natural colour of dark brown instead of the insipid light brown and grey it had become.
I am thrilled with the speed and quality of the results achieved with health kinesiology. Thank you."

Vera Peiffer, London, UK
www.hairgrowthUK.net

Health Kinesiology: Vivian Klein, USA, Case Study

Sonya, married, age 27, had just had a physical because of major symptoms ranging from poor circulation, irregular menstrual cycle, acne, weight gain, high cholesterol, poor liver function and borderline diabetes.

She came to me because the doctor had prescribed so many medications, and she didn't want to pursue that solution to her problems - it felt like covering them up rather than taking care of them. Her eyesight was also beginning to worsen, and she described herself as having become "mean and impatient".

She was living in a very remote part of California because of her husband's work and was pretty cut off from her friends and family. She had been feeling very thirsty at work, but could not drink the spring water from the water cooler - it made her feel ill, so she was drinking distilled water, which did not quench her thirst.

I completed the initial rebalancing of her body and then tested for her body's priority, which was to test the water. She tested allergic to 3 different kinds of water: my well water, bottled spring water and the distilled water as well.

Rather than do the regular HK allergy correction procedure (called symbiotic energy transformation), I did what we call a P/OM. This allows us to "build" a correction tailored to the specific client, when one of the standard techniques just won't do. In this case the body wanted the water samples to be placed on the thymus rather than the usual point near the navel. I did the correction with cosbats (see page 83).

This correction had an immediately profound effect on Sonya. Her mother had driven her to the session, as she did not feel confident to drive. She had entered my therapy room with no energy or life force, looking very pasty and yellow. As she lay on the table and the correction progressed, the color came back into her whole body and even lying down she started remarking that her mind felt clearer.

We did some further psychological corrections in this session to help her adapt to her life in a "little town in the middle of nowhere".

She went home with instructions to drink only a specific brand of bottled water for a few weeks while the energy changes were processed fully by her system. Then she was able to drink any water she wanted. She also had homework: to walk a certain amount of time every week, get to sleep by a certain time every night, and learn to play again (board games and cards with her husband were ok) and also have a separate 'date night' once a week with her husband. All of this was, of course, tested using kinesiology - I didn't just decide what would be good for her.

Sonya came back a month later for a follow up session. She told me she was drinking lots of water. She had lost some weight and was feeling that her life was worth living. She was eating a better diet, was able to exercise and looked bright eyed and rosy instead of yellow and pale.

She was feeling better all around, but had not yet been back to the doctor for retesting. Her acne had started to clear up, and she had had her first menstrual cycle in four months a week after the first session. This continued to be regular during the period of time she was seeing me.

Vivian Klein, California, USA

Health Kinesiology: Deborah Davies & Rebecca Cox, UK, Case Study

Client's story – Rebecca Cox

When I first met Debs, I had identified the various food allergies of my family members through alternative therapies and we were managing them by simply avoiding the foods in question. However, Debs claimed that she could probably 'correct' all of our allergies, so that we would be able to eat everything again without the negative side effects. This was such a bold and assured claim that I had to follow it up.

We have now had four absolutely fascinating HK sessions with Debs, and my family's food allergies - including wheat, dairy, oranges, pulses, chocolate and shellfish - have indeed been entirely corrected.

The sessions are relaxing, interesting and non-invasive, though they are rather unconventional, and you do have to suspend your disbelief as the practitioner converses at length with your arm! The results are so extraordinary that even my husband and more cynical friends have had to accept that HK works - even though none of us understand why.

Debs also identified a number of sources of geopathic stress (see page 35) in our house and my workplace, which she helped me to eliminate. The result of this is that I am sleeping better than I have in years, and my youngest daughter's sleep and behaviour have improved dramatically. Also, with our allergies corrected, we no longer have to seek out alternative foods or be difficult dinner guests. We are now able to eat out as a family, and the children can properly enjoy their friends' birthday parties.

HK has made a huge difference to our lives and - I believe - to our long-term health and well-being. I genuinely could not recommend it more highly, and without a doubt we would turn to it again should any physical, or indeed emotional, issues arise in the future.

Deborah Davies, HK practitioner

When Rebecca and her family first came to me for help with their allergies, I tested (using gentle muscle testing and verbal questioning) to see if I would be able to help them and to establish the best possible way for me to be able to do this for lasting, significant results. It tested up that I would be able to correct their allergies to enable them to eat everything again without the current side effects, which included digestive troubles, fatigue, difficult behavior and bad sleep.

I asked Rebecca if she would like me to correct the identified allergies independently (one by one) or if she would like to me look at the bigger picture. This would include the overall health and wellbeing of the individual and also take into account other stress factors that may have/were contributing to the problems.

She asked me to work with the bigger picture in mind, so that I could ensure the best possible results for overall improved health and happiness.

I then tested to find out the best possible way to help everyone which included the best way to work with them (as a group or individually), the number of sessions needed and how long it would take for them to see improvements. The response was varied - some needed just one session, whereas others needed two. Some of the allergy corrections were done for the whole family with everyone touching one person: they all benefited from the same correction. In all cases it tested that the beneficial results would be instantaneous and that they would then be able to eat the allergens without any problems. I also suggested that at a later point it would be a good idea to look at and address the geopathic stress in the home, which was also having a negative impact on the family's wellbeing. The GS did not test up as a priority, and so we focused on correcting the allergies.

With the young children I used surrogate testing whereby I was able to test and help the child by working on/through the mother. This allowed me to do the HK work without having to directly muscle test the young children or ask them to play an active part in the corrections. Sometimes the children wanted to play an active part; for example, for the allergy tap correction we all tapped the relevant acupuncture points together, which was fun and amusing!

To list all the HK corrections completed over the four sessions would be too lengthy, so here is a summary:

We used a selection of allergy corrections to eliminate the allergens (wheat, dairy, chocolate, soya, pulses, oranges, etc.). These included the allergy tap technique (which enables the body to recognize the allergy substance and respond/process it properly) and the SET allergy detox procedure (which works to thoroughly detoxify the body of the allergen and even other substances holding similar energy patterning while allowing the body to respond appropriately in the future). In HK terms, an allergy is an altered energy response at tissue level as a result of exposure to a substance.

We addressed a number of fears including BBEI's (innate fears set up between conception and first two months), Imperatives (likened to childhood tantrums) and a phobia which focused on 'activity' in the kitchen at home (see below).

We used several Life Transformer Crystals, programmed crystals (see page 42) developed by Dr Jimmy Scott, both in psychological corrections and to wear for a few months following the session (including the one for psychic protection and the one for being centred and grounded). These specially programmed crystals help absorb negative energy patterning from the body while gently reprogramming with appropriate, beneficial patterning.

There are several points which I find of particular interest with this case study, which reinforces my passion for this therapy, its dynamic modalities and ability to get to the source of the problem.

Firstly, although Rebecca came to me confident about her family's allergies, we also discovered that there was a soya allergy. So although they were being very careful to avoid dairy, they had replaced one allergen with another. Because the soya was affecting them in a different way (and not giving them immediate tummy ache reactions), it had not occurred to them that soya might also be detrimental to their health, but it did help explain why the digestive complaints hadn't completely disappeared.

By working with the bigger picture (to significantly improve overall health and wellbeing) not only were we able to identify the soya allergy but also address some of the psychological issues which had developed due to the food allergies, including: having to be the difficult one at school, feeling like the odd one out, not having the freedom to eat with friends and enjoy party food etc.

Having mentioned geopathic stress at the start, it became evident to me during the sessions, that there was also paranormal activity going on in the home as indicated by some of the fears, the phobia and one of the life transformers. Because I felt this was such a strong theme, I gently mentioned it to Rebecca, expecting her to think I was completely mad, but she wasn't at all surprised and even said that she was a little uncomfortable in their home for some reason. It had also become apparent that one of the children was aware of some 'uncomfortable feelings and activity in the kitchen' which she was then able to begin to speak about more openly.

Once we cleared the GS (releasing the spirit of a nurse and closing several energy portals) and in general harmonising the overall energy of the home, the children's behaviour improved, everyone's sleep improved, Rebecca's hair stopped falling out (a symptom that had started soon after they first moved in) and her other allergies disappeared without the need to correct them. This included - champagne, wine and shellfish…her husband, a successful Wine Trader was thrilled!

After the first session, Rebecca commented on how apt and relevant many of the fear corrections had been for the individual children.

Later that day she called me to say that they had eaten cheese on toast for tea, followed by ice cream…and no one had a tummy ache! A week later they were still eating everything and feeling great. A year later they are still eating and enjoying all foods…allergy is a thing of the past, as is the 'nurse' and home really feels like home.

Deborah Davies, Oxfordshire, UK
www.deborahdavies.co.uk

Katrina May (Client of Sandie Lovell), New Zealand writes about Health Kinesiology

I have suffered bouts of depression on and off now for about 12 years and even had an in-patient stint for depression at one of the Priory Clinics while I lived in the UK. I have tried a variety of different therapies from regular counselling to Reiki. They had all helped to some degree, but I continued to feel that there was something blocking my full recovery that I had been unable to shift.

So when my friend told me about Sandie Lovell, I was on the phone the next week to book an appointment. I didn't really know what it was that Sandie did as all my friend had told me was that she didn't have a clue what Sandie was doing, but whatever it was it worked with amazing results! That was enough for me.

In my first consultation Sandie tested and said that I would need 5 sessions over about 12 weeks, which was a welcome change to the normal weekly appointments that can go on for weeks or even months. Apart from dealing with my depression, my goal was to have more energy for parenting and to be able to lighten up and enjoy actively playing with my children. I wanted to wake up feeling zingy!

After one session I had more energy and felt emotionally lighter. I had had some episodes of feeling 'high' with which I felt uncomfortable. I felt that for the first time for 12 years I was over-medicating and a visit to the doctor confirmed this. A blood test ruled out anything else, so the doctor had a chat with the psychiatrist who confirmed over-medication.

My medication was reduced to half the dosage under my doctor's supervision with the result that I felt much more balanced emotionally and didn't experience the uncomfortable 'highs'. By the fifth session, I had more energy in the mornings, enjoyed playing and interacting with the children, and I was down to a quarter of my original medication on alternate days with the goal of coming off it completely.

As I write this I am into my 4th week with no medication! Amazing. I experienced some fairly unpleasant physical withdrawals which I was told would last for about 6 – 8 weeks. After 3 weeks all of these withdrawals disappeared! I feel fantastic mentally. It is a really busy time in our lives and I am ready to take it all on.

I now feel that I have found an alternative option to turn to if I experience another episode of depression, meaning that the doctor and medication can now be a last resort. I am so grateful to have been introduced to Sandie. If anyone asks me what happens in my sessions, my answer is still "I don't really know, she just seems to talk to my arm for an hour but whatever it is she does, I have no doubt that it works."

Katrina May, Wanaka NZ (Practitioner: Sandie Lovell, Wanaka, New Zealand)
www.vitalhealthmatters.com

Integrated Healing

Integrated Healing (IH) was jointly developed by Mathilda van Dyk and Nic Oliver. Mathilda's background is as a psychologist, NLP master practitioner and life coach. Nic's background is as a management development trainer, specialising in leadership development, influencing skills and coaching and NLP master practitioner. He has also been involved in bodywork since 1976, studying anatomy and physiology, biomechanics, kinesiology and exercise physiology, as part of a degree in physical education.

One of the basic concepts of Integrated Healing is that the practitioner does not need to know anything about the disease, trauma or dysfunction that the client comes in with. Everything is seen as being energy with the body manifesting a dysfunction at a particular wavelength and frequency, and, when given the opportunity, it will choose the appropriate frequency to facilitate its healing.

Integrated Healing practitioners do not believe that they heal their clients. Instead, they believe that they are channels to facilitate healing. They create the healing environment, but the healing is carried out by the client's Being. Practitioners strive to ensure that their intent is pure, based on unconditional love for their clients and on doing only what is for the client's highest good.

IH practitioners use a holographic model (see page 31). Healing is seen to be needed on all levels of the person's Being - physical, emotional, mental and spiritual - in order for true healing to take place. By working holographically the practitioner is able to access simultaneously:

- The physical body.
- Feelings and emotions.
- Mental processes, thoughts, values and beliefs.
- Conscious, unconscious and non-conscious processes.
- Imprints and programming.
- Energetic bodies.
- The inner self.
- The soul/higher self.

Integrated Healing sees the session as a healing pathway reflecting the journey from a dysfunctional state to a healed state. At the beginning of an IH session some standard kinesiology pre-tests are carried out, e.g. switching (see page 33), hydration, etc. There is a protocol template that allows practitioners to work with any issue presented to them by the client. Built in safety checks minimise the chances of healing crises occurring.

Integrated Healing practitioners use both binary (see page 15) and holographic muscle testing (see page 15). For holographic muscle testing, practitioners often use the shoulder group of muscles to give a percentage display. 100% is when the arm is perpendicular to the body, and

0% is when the arm is beside the body. IH practitioners use finger modes (see page 21), or verbal statements (not verbal questions). An analogy is that on a computer desktop you have icons (equivalent to finger modes) and the text label underneath (verbal statements in IH).

Integrated Healing makes extensive use of adding to circuit (see page 20). Scan lists are used to find all the information related to the issue being worked on. Correcting procedures include hands on healing techniques involving the aura (see page 13), chakras (see page 08), meridians, extra vessels, dantians, assemblage point, etc. Practitioners are not limited to only using IH correction procedures but are free to offer any healing correction they know, with the specific correction determined by muscle testing. Neuro-Linguistic Programming (NLP) techniques (such as anchoring, reframing and mental imagery, etc.) may also be used. NLP 'tools-for-change' are used to ensure that the client creates a clearly defined outcome and that the client owns their healed state. IH also integrates insights from Cognitive Behavioural Therapy and Life Coaching.

IH practitioners often address issues such as self-sabotage, inappropriate survival programs, inner child healing, soul integration, deep level neurological switching, negative amygdala memories, inappropriate energetic ties, self-limiting beliefs, phobias, etc. IH practitioners use simple protocols to deal with these issues and find that in working holographically many chronic symptoms disappear.

www.integratedhealing.co.uk

Mathilda Van Dyk, UK, talking about Integrated Healing

I used to be a psychologist but became increasingly frustrated by the limitations of talk therapies; I was then introduced to kinesiology. I did over 60 courses and sometimes I thought: "Wow, this is great stuff, but why does it have to be so long-winded, so complicated?" Other times I felt positive about the course but had a nagging feeling that I wanted something different.

For example, sometimes I'd get iffy muscle testing, the muscle felt "spongy" rather than giving a definite response and I knew the Being was trying to tell me something, but I didn't know what. So I started to rant at the Universe - at least, that's what Nic* called it! Then answers and eventually whole protocols started to come through. I asked for a safe, guided, easy way of working with the whole being; and it had to be simple. I wasn't thinking that I was going to teach - I just wanted it for myself and for my clients.

Even though I'd asked for it to be simple, when we started writing the manuals, we kept catching ourselves complicating it, to give it more "substance", to make it more "impressive". But we realised that we needed to keep it clear and beautiful to retain its essence, its spirit. So we did that, but then as time went on, we started complicating it again. It took a broken jaw to make me get the message from the Universe once and for all.

I was visiting my family, just returning from having wiring and implants in my jaw; my face was all bruised and swollen. My three year old nephew said he wanted to pray to make it better. Then he said he could make it better by putting his hand there. This kid had attended no courses, used no structures, just total purity and love. (And nobody told him that healing couldn't be that easy!) The next day I was back eating cornflakes.** All the pain, swelling and most of the bruising was gone. We talked to him about what he did, and he explained it like this: "I looked and put my hands where they needed to go; I asked Jesus to make it better; I waited for the love to flow; then I said thank you." He used Jesus because his mother is a pastor, so that was his frame of reference. Although IH has a strong spiritual foundation, we welcome people from all religions and those who aren't religious at all.

We started sharing our work with other kinesiologists, first in England, then in Australia - now IH has spread to more than twenty countries on six continents. I was really nervous at first, because the system was so simple, but other kinesiologists, many of them with over 20 years of kinesiology experience, really liked it, and appreciated its simplicity.

I love the holographic approach; we don't focus on just clearing symptoms. There is an ancient Chinese saying which can be summed up as: "Don't heal the disease, heal the whole person." We frequently meet healers who are confident about working on a sprained ankle, but worry about working with a more "challenging" condition such as severe arthritis. Our interpretation of the Chinese saying is that IH practitioners never need to worry about working with a disease that they may not even know anything about. To us, every dysfunction/disease is just an energetic blockage expressed as a frequency. Our intent is to create an environment where the client's Being feels safe, and where it will reveal the opposite frequency to the dysfunction. We can then introduce that frequency into the body and their condition will 'collapse' and healing will take place.

A lot of IH is channelled; I wake in the night and write things down. In the morning, Nic deciphers my handwriting and we then work with it. Then we give it to research kinesiologists to work with, before it makes its way into the IH manuals. Nic writes all the manuals as he's been writing manuals of one sort or another for over twenty five years.

A central concept is soul integration. I was really dismissive of the idea that there may be fragments of a person's soul somewhere out there in the Universe, and you first have to bring them home. Nic bought Sandra Ingerman's book on soul retrieval work. He went to Brussels and read it at the airport and in the hotel. That evening he told me on the phone that he thought it was important stuff, as Ingerman's view is that 'change can only work on the parts that are at home', and that he would tell me more about it when he came home. I was still dismissive. I went to bed, woke up in the middle of the night and wrote down the complete soul integration protocol. There were very clear instructions that we should call it soul integration and not soul retrieval. (Soul retrieval requires shamanic journeying, which we don't do. Soul integration uses a model where part of the soul has ceased to communicate with the rest but now needs re-integrating.) When Nic came home, he told me he'd also written one. When we compared them, they were 80% the same. That gave us immense confidence that we had something special.

We don't force anything on anyone. We start with a generic protocol looking at where you are and where you want to be. We use holographic recording, so it's not just a snapshot of a dysfunction, but a full colour video. For example, if someone came to me with problems with their golf swing, I'd ask them to bring their golf clubs with them. I'd get the person to perform the golf swing while I used holographic recording. That way we get all the different stressful aspects of the golf swing, including the anatomical stressors, neurological issues, anything emotional such as memories of an old injury or fear of a new injury, self-limiting beliefs, etc. - whatever is relevant to the problem.

If people have emotional issues they don't even have to talk about it; all they need to do is think about the issue while the practitioner does holographic recording of the impact of the issue on the client's total being. Sometimes that is enough to work with; it's like removing a tree that's fallen into a stream. But sometimes it's the bigger picture that needs looking at; the whole mountain that the tree grew on has fallen into the stream, and the 'tree' is just a symptom. When that happens, the client's Being will guide us to look for deep seated root cause issues such as sabotage programs, inner child issues, deep level neurological switching, negative amygdala programs, soul integration, self-limiting beliefs, energetic cords and many more.

We always challenge using muscle testing to make sure we have enough information. Some people don't have a frame of reference that includes chakras or soul integration etc. and for those people, testing probably won't bring it up. But we never make assumptions. Every step of our protocol is always determined by muscle testing, and we are totally guided by the wisdom of the client's Being, we work at a level that each person is ready to accept, that reflects what they can handle. This is one of the reasons why we don't have healing crises in IH.

In IH we trust the Power that created the being to heal the being. Healing comes from the heart and by making the process simple, practitioners can get out of their heads and into their hearts to facilitate gentle and profound healings. I love the work I do and am passionate about sharing it with other people around the world.

Mathilda van Dyk, UK
www.integratedhealing.co.uk

* Nic Oliver is Mathilda's husband and co-developer of Integrated Healing.
** 'Cornflakes' is a crunchy breakfast cereal.

Keita Saito, Yukino Saito and Hiroaki Nishida, Japan, talking about Integrated Healing

Keita Saito:
I was originally a chiropractor but sometimes cures didn't happen. I found kinesiology as a hope for my sessions.

I studied other kinesiologies first. Then I found Integrated Healing. I had been using muscle testing without any real understanding, but after training in IH I knew specifically what I was doing and could clearly understand the answers given to me through the muscle testing. I really liked the IH pathway system of chakras. It's very special to me. I find IH simple but profound. I like working in the holographic way, not just testing locked/unlock, but testing inter-connections. I used to focus on the physical body dealing with structure. I have always been interested in other aspects, but I didn't know how to integrate them into what I do. I do very little chiropractic now, maybe 5 or 6 times a year, when the client's body says it needs it.

Megumi (not her real name) was a depressive. A friend had committed suicide. He had made a time- bomb, strapped it to himself, and then it went off automatically killing him. Megumi had had to clean the room afterwards. I found that Megumi had a strong psychic attack from her friend who had died. I used IH protocols to deal with that. I want to emphasise that Megumi got better after that - just one session, and her husband who was also depressed got better after he had a session. During the session tears flowed from my eyes; I felt no emotions - no sadness, no anger - the tears just flowed. That was the remarkable thing about that session, and I still remember it clearly.

Another client lost half her eyelashes – one day, about three years ago, they suddenly fell out and didn't regrow. After our session more fell out the next day! Her session protocol was the blueprint. Muscle testing showed her theme was that she wanted to train to be an instructor for the basic kinesiology course, but she wasn't confident enough to do it. I found that this was because of how her teacher was in the first ever kinesiology course she had taken. Because her first experience of kinesiology was so difficult, she kept finding in her heart that teaching kinesiology was difficult. She cried a lot during the session and had vivid dreams that night, but she realised that she could be a basic kinesiology instructor if she wanted to do it, but she also realised that she didn't want to do it. By the way her eyelashes also regrew and have stayed.

I used to feel tired a lot after sessions, but now with Integrated Healing this is much less. Learning Integrated Healing has given me enough confidence to say I am a professional kinesiologist.

Yukino Saito:
Doing Integrated Healing is my life work. Before I was doing so many things - homeopathy, hypnotherapy, flower essences, aromatherapy. I could not feel real satisfaction with each of them, so I was looking for something else. With IH I can use everything I have learnt in the best way for the client at that moment. Within the IH framework I can use everything, including anything new I learn.

I like the way IH treats clients in a holographic way. For example, if someone has a pain in the back, we deal with the pain in the back and the emotions and the environment - anything that is important in that moment.

I had a client with a phobia of entering an express train. At one time Keiko (not her real name) could do it, but when she was 20 she became afraid. Her boyfriend suffered from a panic disorder and started to scream and tremble. This happened in his flat, but afterwards Keiko stopped being able to board an express train. The IH protocol Cutting Energetic Cords came up. Naturally I supposed it was to the boyfriend, but testing showed it was with her father. Keiko told me they loved each other, and that there were no negative cords to cut. So, we looked further and it showed that her father loved her so much he didn't want to let her go. Afterwards I went with Keiko to the express train. Before getting into the train, she started crying. I asked her if the phobia was still there, but she told me that she was remembering how afraid she had been and she was feeling pity for her old self. She no longer has the phobia.

When we had the session, Keiko was no longer with the boyfriend and had since been married and divorced from another man. Now, since the session, she has a new boyfriend and is very happy. Keiko says that before the session she always had problems in her relationship with men, and she thinks that was because of this strong energy from her father. She also thinks that the express train symbolized going away from her father.

Hiroaki Nishida, who also helped me as interpreter for Yukino and Keita:
When I came for my first session, I knew that I had many problems –money, home, parents. Muscle checking showed that money was the issue for the session. It showed that I'm too in my head, so that I cannot act. The goal setting for the session was: "I will buy an expensive shirt feeling expanded like a blue shining sky". The relevant protocol was Inner Child and was for one month after my conception. At that time my inner child was enclosing itself and withdrawing. The grown up me wanted to use money, but my inner child was preoccupied with saving money; the inner child was still driving me to make too much effort to save money. The inner child message was to tell my father that it is OK to receive the results of your effort without guilt. This message meant that if you have money it is OK; you do not need to get rid of it as quickly as possible. My inner child and unconscious was satisfied. We used some cranial osteopathy as part of the correcting procedure. Keita found the left and right cranial bones were very different and were affecting the brainstem. Muscle testing showed that while my mother was pregnant she was saving a lot, but my father was just spending money. We used Tibetan bells and another osteopathic technique. The 6th chakra needed support from the energy of an eight star diamond. These diamonds have high optical symmetry and are vibrationally different from other diamonds. We read some information on these diamonds and then closed the session.

Before the session I always had difficulty sustaining living even though I worked hard and struggled a lot. Now I can sustain living and business sometimes comes to me without any effort on my part.

www.kinesiology.co.jp
www.kinesiology-seminar.com

Integrated Healing: Marisa Russo, Australia, Case Study
Karla's mother treated her differently from her other siblings. She was very cold and hard towards her. Her father scolded her regularly. Karla felt she did not fit in. Because of her red hair and blue eyes, Karla suspected she was the result an unwanted pregnancy from a family relative.

As a child, Karla's parent put her to work on the farm where they lived when she returned home from school. She felt she was treated differently from her other siblings as they seem to get away with more than she did. She felt her siblings seemed to have less judgments and punishments put on them from her parents. She was also sexually abused by a family friend. Her mother screamed, laying the blame on her even though she was only 7 years of age. Life really seemed cruel.

As she grew older and became an adult her life continued in the same manner with abusive and destructive relationships. Karla felt very 'shattered' and lost.

When I began the 'Soul Integration' protocol, Karla started to feel overwhelmed. I could sense the energy begin to form in the room to prepare Karla for what was about to take place. I was grateful for the first step in the protocol which includes "divine protection". Divine protection sets up the protocol so that there is assistance from divine sources to protect you and the client while you work together. When you are dealing with big traumas and abuse, this can be overwhelming for the client, and it can lead to a 'healing crisis'. Asking for divine protection limits the negative consequences and repercussions for the client.

It took some time for me to work through each step. Each step is devised so that you need a confirmation or the go ahead to move on. This ensures enough information and support for the client has been obtained so that the outcome is satisfactorily reached. The longer the protocol takes the more assistance and energy is needed; long protocols often means that you are dealing with deep seated issues. Integrated Healing provides a flow chart to select which correction or energy is needed; this makes a profound healing still simple to follow. When I reached the step in the protocol for Karla to repeat the statement: "I, Karla, now release all the stressful negative memories that caused my soul to fracture", Karla burst into tears. For a moment she felt the pain of her soul fragments shattering in all her trauma. Karla explained it felt like a few seconds of sharp pain in her heart, as if it resembled the emotional pain she endured when she was a child.

As I continued to work through the protocol of integrating the fragments, which is a process of requesting retrieval of the fragments and then requesting for the fragments to be integrated. Stillness came over the room and her body. I then tested for her soul message which was: "It is ok to allow someone else to care for you". As I told Karla this, a smile came over her face. Karla said that for the first time in her life she felt whole. She said she now felt that she deserved love. She then shed tears of joy as she lay in peace on the treatment couch.

Karla now says that since that session she feels a deep peace inside her herself and that the need to look for love outside herself has diminished. It has assisted her with feeling whole and more connected to people. It has given peace to her traumatised and fragmented soul.

Marisa Russo, Melbourne, Australia
www.marisarusso.com

A Client Of Practitioner Tamlyn Hill, USA, writing about Integrated Healing

I was first introduced to Integrated Healing when I began searching for a way to manage and control my scattered and unfocused thoughts, mounting frustrations and constant feelings of irritation and agitation. Emotional, physical and spiritual changes happened very quickly during and after the first session. It was then than I began to realize that unpleasant childhood memories had greatly impacted me more than I had ever imagined. This revelation explains the years of feeling inadequate, lacking self-esteem, self-confidence and never truly feeling comfortable with myself.

Addressing issues relating to my childhood helps shed light on a lifetime of ingrained behavioural patterns. Each session allows me the opportunity to look at myself and face my fears truthfully no matter how hard and painful this may be. Seeing the truth has been liberating and has set me free in so many ways. An entire new world has opened up for me, and I am seeing life from a new, different and refreshing perspective. I have learned to cherish and embrace change, taking ownership and responsibility for my own personal growth and development, physical wellness, emotional well-being, spirituality and happiness.

Integrated Healing has changed my entire thought process and the way that I view everything. Negative thoughts and self-doubts that used to dominate my mind are but a distant memory and have been replaced by a quiet yet strong inner strength, and the courage to step out and have confidence and faith while enjoying the journey. My spirituality has deepened immensely and is now at the center of everything that I do. Emotions that once were embedded and trapped so deep in the subconscious mind have risen to the surface and a multitude of thoughts and feelings have been extracted and revelations glaringly exposed. Having been taken to levels so deep emotionally, there is now an overall and continual self-awareness that was not present ever before. These self-discoveries have been stunning and shocking and the results incredible and amazing.

Integrated Healing has been an absolutely phenomenal life-changing experience. True healing and deep soul-searching have taken place on all levels: emotionally, physically and spiritually. I no longer feel agitated, irritated or frustrated. My overall mind-set and outlook have shifted completely in addition to experiencing incredible energy shifts. One of the biggest and most dramatic changes that has occurred has been the gradual progression of truly being comfortable and secure with the person that I have become, and liking and loving myself in the process.

Previously unrecognizable self-imposed beliefs have limited my growth as a person all of these years, but, because of newfound self-esteem and self-confidence, I am seeing and now tapping into my true potential. More importantly, these overall changes have led to a change for the better as a human being, and for this I am most grateful and thankful. The personal transformations have been astonishing and remarkable. I have been enlightened in countless ways and have a profound sense of joy, happiness and purpose along with an inner calmness, peace and balance that never existed previously.

I feel extremely fortunate that a "partnership" formed during the Integrated Healing sessions with my practitioner, Tamlyn Hill. We have connected on an entirely different level which has allowed incredible changes to occur. My heart and mind have been open to receiving anything and everything from her, and Tamlyn's heart is always centered in the right place. It is important that I unequivocally state that none of these profound personal transformations would have been possible or would have taken place without Tamlyn, who puts her heart and soul into each of our sessions. One can't help but feed off of someone who possesses incredible energy, a genuinely loving and giving spirit, and a superior and extraordinary intuitive nature. An undeniable and infectious radiance always surrounds Tamlyn, and that sphere extends outwardly to all of her clients. I have an indescribable gratitude to Tamlyn who masterfully weaves and incorporates Integrated Healing into our sessions. I feel so richly blessed to be in the presence of such a beautiful person who exudes love, warmth, patience, kindness, passion and compassion.

I truly believe Integrated Healing is a gift that must be shared with everyone, and both clients and practitioners must dutifully pass on this infinite gift to all those individuals who cross our paths.

Written by a client of practitioner Tamlyn Hill, Colorado, USA
www.soaringspiritinstitute.com

Integrated Healing: Tabitha Gale, UK, Case Study

Jenny (not her real name) came to see me suffering with stomach ache, bloating and wind, (which her GP had diagnosed as irritable bowel syndrome). Jenny, who was in her thirties, had been careful with what she was eating and had tried leaving things out of her diet, but this had not helped. As a result there was a lot of anxiety around eating and she would comfort eat at times. Jenny was taking anti-depressants, which her doctor had prescribed to try and lessen the comfort eating. She now wanted to stop taking these and replace them with a more natural approach, if possible.

During her first session with me, Jenny chose a full Reiki session. As often happens, whilst giving Reiki I sensed that her energy field was offering me some information, which I passed on to Jenny to see what it meant to her. The phrases I was given were: 'life's a struggle', and 'a psychological battle is going on'. As a consequence, Jenny talked about her relationship with her mother and father, both of whom she found unsupportive in relation to the line of work she wished to pursue. She said she was distressed doing a job that she did not like. There was a lot of stress around this subject, so we did Emotional Stress Release (ESR, see page 40), whilst she thought about how she could better deal with her parents – and she came up with great solutions. I also did Reiki healing around her stomach area, known as the solar plexus energy centre.

At Jenny's second session she told me she had had no symptoms of IBS since our first meeting. Under the guidance of her GP, she was now taking fewer anti-depressants and was hoping to finish taking them altogether by the end of the next month. She had found a new job and wished to use this session to work on preparing herself calmly to manage the challenges of this new role.

We decided to do an Integrated Healing balance for this second session, the main corrections for which were Reiki healing, mostly on her left side. We also focused energy into her kidney points on the soles of the feet (a good energy boost). We then checked whether Jenny needed any support to help with her balance, so far. Muscle testing pinpointed a statement from the Raw Affirmation Book, which read: 'I release ......'s energies. I am my own person and am responsible for me only'. Jenny responded to this by saying she felt that her parents were pulling on her emotions, even when she was away from them. We checked again (using muscle monitoring) and found there was indeed an energetic connection (energetic cords) to feelings that belonged to her parents, rather than herself. These were affecting her energy levels and emotional feelings. We cleared these using Reiki and visualisation (see page 39), and re-checked that we had successfully cleared them afterwards.

No foods showed up as being a problem for Jenny, and she reported feeling much lighter and relaxed afterwards.

When Jenny came for her final appointment, her goal was to maintain good energy levels and work-life balance to help her train for the Race for Life, a five kilometre charity run. She had finished her course of anti-depressants and said she was feeling fine without them. A final message from her energy field in this session was 'self acceptance without judgment'. We again used ESR with this as the focus - ESR can be used for future events, performance and changing behaviours - while Jenny visualised being less hard on herself and generally more self-accepting and supportive of herself.

This is a beautiful example of how when we get in touch with what is really going on for us, not just emotionally and physically, but in the context of our lives, changes can happen fast - not only in our bodies, but with our journey in life. When we set ourselves on the right track, the path that is right for us and the right opportunities seem to appear. Once Jenny had released the stress that had built up around her circumstance of being in the wrong job, and torn about leaving because this was not her parents wish for her, she became clear about the direction she wished to go in and had a great offer of a job she wanted. We were then able to clear the feelings and energies that had been holding her back, enabling her to move freely in the direction she wished.

Tabitha Gale, Bristol, England
www.bristolkinesiology.co.uk

Kinergetics

Philip Rafferty of Australia became a full-time kinesiology practitioner in 1988 after studying various branches of kinesiology. Philip had also experienced the benefits of Reiki healing and decided to channel healing into the organ associated with an unlocked muscle. He found that unlocked muscles then tested locked. In 1991 he established Kinergy, (the name changed to Kinergetics in 1995) a combination of muscle testing and Reiki healing. He started to teach it but soon found that students needed to learn Reiki healing first. He looked for a way of switching on healing energy without the need for Reiki training. He realised that everyone is able to heal, but it may be necessary to clear the blocks to allow the practitioner's natural healing potential to manifest.

Kinergetics practitioners see the energy system as storing memories of everything that has happened throughout life - experiences, traumas, thoughts, emotions, relationships, etc. Pain, disease and psychological problems occur because of blocks in the subtle energy field caused by these past events. The practitioner works to clear these blockages, so that the body's ability to heal itself can be activated and encouraged.

Muscle testing is used to identify the area of pain or imbalance and to find exactly where the correction is needed. Corrections involve channelling energy through the hands usually to muscles, organs, glands or chakras. The practitioner may touch the client while this is being done, through clothing where appropriate, or else may hold the hands off the body at a precise point determined by muscle testing.

Kinergetics practitioners make extensive use of scan lists to assess a client for sensitivities, emotions (420 of them), hydration problems, temporomandibular joint imbalances (TMJ, see page 34) hypertonic muscles, priority imbalance, chakras, etc.

Jaw stacking (see page 20) is used to store all the information and imbalances that are accessed before healing can take place.

Hydration balancing is an important feature of Kinergetics and is seen to correct many other imbalances. Hydration corrections do not necessarily involve drinking water; the client may not be drinking water because they have difficulty in using it properly and so feel bloated when they drink a normal amount. Emotional or biochemical stress can cause problems for the kidneys and other organs, so they function less well. Kinergetics practitioners find that every new client requires the Kinergetics hydration balance. Hydration balancing has been found to be particularly important and beneficial for chronic pain, but can also make a dramatic and lasting difference to a whole range of other problems.

Kinergetics practitioners also see a link between dehydration and TMJ problems: improving hydration will reduce TMJ imbalances, and a good TMJ correction will improve hydration. If the TMJ is out of balance, the sphenoid (a bone at the base of the skull) is also out of balance. This affects the person's physical balance and also the pituitary gland, which is the master gland co-ordinating the activity of all the other hormone producing glands. So, a TMJ problem can lead to a hormone imbalance.

Hydration and TMJ imbalances can lead to other problems too, including problems with mineral absorption and learning difficulties. Many Kinergetics sessions will start with rebalancing these two problem areas.

Using scan lists, age recession (see page 39) and muscle testing the practitioner is able to pinpoint the age at which the problem started and the key emotions that were involved at that time. Through the Kinergetics work the client is able to let go of old pains and traumas, whether conscious or otherwise, and approach life with a new and more positive outlook.

Allergies are often seen to be connected to a trauma or unpleasant experience in the past, causing an often unconscious reaction to that experience which manifests as an allergic reaction. By healing the negative energy associated with the experience, the allergy can also be removed, so the Kinergetics practitioner seeks to find the emotional trigger and work with that. Practitioners also work extensively with Candida problems and heavy metal problems.

There are several TMJ corrections within Kinergetics, but Philip also developed RESET (Rafferty Energy System of Easing the Temporomandibular joint). This is taught as a completely separate workshop. TMJ corrections involve re-balancing the muscles around the jaw. In RESET this is done by sending healing energy into the muscles and tendons that relate to the TMJ, which not only affects the TMJ itself but also other associated muscles, bones, organs and glands.

www.kinergetics.com.au
www.reset-tmj.com

Philip Rafferty, Australia, talking about Kinergetics

I first got interested in Touch for Health and did a basic Touch for Health course in 1981. I wanted to learn more, but there weren't any courses locally, so I phoned the US office and went to America to learn more and become a TFH instructor. If I want something, I just go for it! Then I started organising courses and bringing kinesiology teachers over to Australia. I was working in restaurants at the time, and couldn't always get the time off. When that happened, I just left the job and then found another job after the course.

Over time I developed my own kinesiology system - Kinergetics. Kinergetics is a fast, non-invasive, simple, effective method of releasing pain and stress and locating and correcting some of the emotional and metaphysical causes of disease. In Kinergetics we obtain feedback about the state of the meridians in the body through muscle testing. Meridians are an intricate part of a whole network of 'circuits' interconnecting different parts and functions of the body. When these circuits are disturbed, problems result.

A lot of kinesiology systems have many different corrections to correct these problems, but Kinergetics only has one - the use of healing energy - this can correct almost any circuit. Usually in Kinergetics we load different things into the circuit and then perform the one correction at the end. You can load information about the causes of imbalances. The Kinergetics practitioner may scan lists or use test kits to find the necessary emotions or blocks they need to add in before they do the correction.

First we check 16 muscles, using the standard 14 muscles (see page 17) that most kinesiologies use, plus sartorius (for the adrenals) and middle trapezius (for the spleen).

We balance the TMJ (see page 34) and check hydration (see page 35) first because they affect so much – the whole energy system is affected and both TMJ and hydration affect kidney energy. Finding and correcting the stresses that block the assimilation of water will very often correct 95% of muscles in the body. Some people don't drink any water because they can't utilise it, they just feel bloated. Obviously they get water from food, but once the blocks to assimilation are corrected they start drinking water. At the other extreme, one boy was drinking eight litres a day - and had major problems. After a basic hydration correction he reduced to two litres a day.

Correcting assimilation of water and the TMJ gives a really solid structural and energetic foundation to the work. We then retest the 16 muscles. If there's still a muscle out of balance, (which is rarely) we load in more information and correct that.

We also specialise in balancing candida and heavy metals, sabotages and stress, and have a reputation for helping really difficult cases. One example was a lady who came in with chronic head pain and said: "If you touch my neck I will vomit." She left pain free, with no vomiting. Another lady had severely deformed hands and was in chronic pain. Using a metals test kit, I found a severe energetic reaction to platinum. She wore a metal watch and lived in a country that uses platinum in catalytic converters in cars. Months later I received an email that she was still pain-free. Even difficult cases like multiple sclerosis, chronic fatigue and fibromyalgia are often helped.

The new Master Class has an incredibly fast Trauma Balance. I have now balanced over 1,000 traumas, most in less than five minutes. It changes clients' reaction to trauma – one client described it as now having bullet-proof glass in front of the trauma.

I developed the system in 1991, and since then kinergetics has been successful in helping thousands of people in over 20 countries. It is particularly good for easing pain as it accesses so many different causes - structural, emotional, energetic and spiritual. Unit 1, the basic two-day workshop, has three very powerful pain corrections.

I have done over 100 demonstrations in 17 countries. I ask for volunteers with the highest level of pain first, or the biggest trauma. In the short demonstrations about 80% of people in pain or trauma notice significant improvement. The Kinergetics website has over 300 testimonials.

I love doing free demonstrations and travel to Europe most years!

Philip Rafferty, Tasmania, Australia
www.reset-tmj.com
www.kinergetics.com.au

Tawni K. Lawrence, USA, writing about Kinergetics

I have been using Kinergetics for years to assist with hydration issues both with myself and with clients. I have seen great results from this work. I have found if the body is hydrated it allows me to go deeper into the body to heal the system. When the body feels supported with its hydration, it will reveal more blockages.

I had an amazing experience. I was receiving a balance by two veteran kinesiologists. It was a big issue and I could feel that energetically I was out in the energy fields – it felt safe being detached. The more they worked with their tools to get me "present", the more I knew I wasn't going to co-operate. Finally, I thought to do a Kinergetics "hydration balance" on myself. I have witnessed the effects of this great work on other people, I have felt better after I received the work, but I have NEVER felt what I felt with this. The MINUTE my mind/body/spirit were energetically hydrated I was totally connected. I can't put into words how present I instantly became, how good I felt, and the shift I had.

On another occasion I had my blood drawn for a live blood analysis. The practitioner told me my red blood cells were dehydrated because they were sticking together. He started to tell me of all the things I would have to do when I returned home. I asked him to wait ten minutes and let me go into another room where I would give myself a Kinergetics hydration balance; then I would be back for another blood draw. He was amazed when he saw my red blood cells after the 10-minute energetic hydration correction. Actually, I was amazed, too. They were flowing freely.

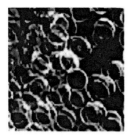   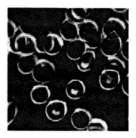

Before Correction   After Correction

Philip Rafferty, creator of Kinergetics (one of many branches of energy kinesiology), has created a protocol which allows one to find and energetically release blockages that prohibits the absorption and utilization of water. Heather was living in Japan when she got mercury poisoning. She returned to the States, spent a year doing every traditional method she could to heal, then resorted to alternative methods. Some things were improving but her kidneys were just not sloughing off the mercury, and her doctor told her she was weeks away from kidney dialysis.

Through muscle checking, Philip found Heather's kidneys to be energetically dehydrated. Her kidneys just did not have the support they needed to slough off the mercury. He did a 20-minute balance (a process to bring the body into homeostasis) which assisted her body in clearing the dehydration blockages. The turnaround was amazing. Her kidneys had the support they needed to release the mercury. She is now healthy and has since had two children.

I use Kinergetics all the time along with many other modalities. I appreciate the depth of this work and all its many facets.

Tawni K. Lawrence, Sandy, Utah, USA
www.kinergetics.com.au/PracDetail.asp?UserID=96

Kinergetics: Natalie G. Nehman, USA, Case Study

This is a case history of the mother of an Energy Kinesiology (EnK) student in New York State. Since I teach several different branches of EnK, Naomi (not her real name) was quite familiar with many of the techniques that I use. When appropriate, I discuss various experiences to show how the technique can be used. Naomi felt that I could help her mother with a problem she had had for some seven months.

Naomi's mother, Barbara (not her real name), had been treated several times for E.coli in her bladder. She had been experiencing overall weakness as well as strange sensations in the bladder area. She also told me that it felt like the E. coli was on the outside of her bladder. (A very strange thing to say, I thought, but took note.) Having had ten children with some still home in need of care, Barbara was anxious to get her energy back and to be feeling better.

As both Naomi and her mother explained, she had already completed two rounds of antibiotics. Both times she had waited the prescribed time for the antibiotics to be effective and then had gone for retesting, only to find that the E.coli was still there. The third antibiotic caused an allergic reaction that sent her to the hospital for about 10 days. As the fourth and fifth antibiotic did not clear the E.coli out of her bladder, Barbara asked the doctor what he would do next. When he said: "more antibiotics", Barbara said: "No! I'm going to go see a natural therapist, Natalie, and try that instead."

After getting an idea of the issue, it seemed logical that the best place to start was to use a protocol on micro-organisms with her. This comes from Kinergetics. I have always had good success with it. I explained that I couldn't guarantee her the desired results any more than her doctor could. But because of my past experience with this technique, I thought there was a good chance that she would be free of her problem but I wanted her to let me know after she had her blood and urine tests again.

In Kinergetics it is always recommended that we hydrate the body first, before we work on the issue at hand. That will allow the body to do its own healing better: the water and nutrients can get into the relevant cells, and the dead cells and debris can get out. This is an energetic balance done using muscle monitoring.

I then went to the micro-organism scan chart to see which micro-organism, if any, was the priority to work on. Although it seemed likely that we would be working with the E. Coli bacteria, it is always important to check and not just make an assumption. The muscle monitoring responses allow her body to communicate with mine. We always use finger modes (see page 21) and jaw stacking (see page 20), as we build large circuits (files) to clear out what her body 'says' needs attention. In the case of micro-organisms, Philip Rafferty (the founder of Kinergetics) has found that the facilitator needs to lower her energy to match that of the micro-organism (as in homeopathy, like neutralizes like), when sending the energy to where the client's body needed it most. (Normally we would raise our energy to a higher level during a session.)

At the end of this protocol we always check the bladder and bladder wall and balance those with energy. (Energetic imbalances seem to detoxify primarily through the bladder.) Because of her strange statement about 'outside the bladder', I also added that into the protocol for her. At this point a Kinergetics practitioner will always check to see if it is safe to close the circuit or not and handle that. We do not want the client to have a healing crisis when it can probably be avoided at this point. We will end the session by checking the client's hydration again and also their electrolytes (dissolved minerals.) These will be energetically balanced as well, so that the client's body will be in the best shape possible to handle what we just did.

Several weeks later when I heard from Barbara she was so excited. She explained that the day after our session together she had had a very, very strange feeling in her body and then knew that the E.coli in her bladder was gone. She also reported that finally after more than eight months and five antibiotics her medical tests showed that after our session together the E.coli was in reality gone. Her energy was back, her strange sensations were gone, her sleeping was better, and she felt she was functioning like her old self again! I was so happy for her.

Natalie G. Nehman, Florida, USA
www.balancingbasics.com

Kinesiología Psicoenergética

Juan Carlos Monge, Spain, talking about Kinesiología Psicoenergética

My first contact with kinesiology was when I was seventeen. I had met a chiropractor from the USA, and he demonstrated some very basic stuff. I didn't understand what it was, but later when I got involved in kinesiology I realised that it was Touch for Health. I was doing yoga and other things at the time, having fun, but I lost contact with the chiropractor.

I really got involved in all this stuff at the end of the 80's, beginning of the 90's. I went to a demonstration organised by a natural products company, and one of the presenters started to show some kinesiology. Francesca Simeon, my partner, and I just felt we needed to know more: Is it fake? Is it true? Does it work?

We started researching kinesiology and found kinesiologists in other parts of Spain, so we started bringing them in for kinesiology workshops. After about two years we started travelling abroad to courses and international conferences in order to learn more. We also started to bring in people from outside Spain: Andrew Verity, John and Matthew Thie, Charles Krebs, Philip Rafferty, Bruce Dewe, Gordon Stokes and Daniel Whiteside - lots of different people.

Things were growing and growing and about 1994 we decided to be fully devoted to kinesiology. Francesca was a clinical psychologist and I was an osteopath and physiotherapist, but we had found that kinesiology helped us the most with our own health so we decided to focus on that. All the teaching was focussed on kinesiology, and 90 to 95% of what we did in our clinic was kinesiology too. Kinesiology gives you a framework that allows you to move very comfortably and to respect the client and respect all the tools you use.

At the end of the 90's -1998- we organised an international kinesiology conference in Spain. We realised we wanted to offer a basic kinesiology training for people, and then advanced courses from different people and different kinesiology systems - a wide approach, not just focussing on one kinesiology.

In 2005 the Catalan government set out to regulate natural therapies, so we presented a programme setting out content and competencies. But the law was not completed in the end. Since then we've had contact with universities, and one university, Real Centro Universitario Maria Cristina, endorses our training, so people can get a diploma. Students come to our school and get the training here, theoretical and practical. At the end they go to the university and have the final assessment there. So they get the University accreditation. There are 3 kinds of diplomas - 1 year, 2 year and 4 year. The four year training is a private University Degree in Complementary Health Therapies, speciality Kinesiología Psicoenergética. We coined the term Kinesiologia Psicoenergetica, as it is not Academic Kinesiology. Also, as people study the various advanced courses, they can get certificates from the different kinesiology systems.

In 1998 we were still organising all our activities from a small place; it just wasn't big enough. We wanted something bigger. So we made this stupid decision to make a kinesiology school!! We focussed on what we wanted to create - the building we want, the recognition for the college we want, what sort of project it is… We started in 1998; we set up goals, set up different facets; we set up the energy. We kept giving each other balances for that. We found some land close to Barcelona and went to the town council to get planning permission for our college. That was no problem. Then we went to the bank to get a loan. We were asked: how many kinesiology colleges are there in Spain? How can you ask for all this money? We asked lots of different banks, but they all turned us down. One bank suggested we should change the name of the school, pretend we were doing psychology and physiotherapy because of our earlier training, but we refused - kinesiology is what we do!

During a seminar we started talking about what we wanted to do and the problems we were having. One student said: let's do a goal setting and a group defusion. So we did this with the whole class connected together and using one person as the surrogate (see page 18). Then just before she left, one of the ladies said: I've just remembered - I have a friend that works in a bank. The very next day we had an appointment with this person and a week later we had the credit - nobody gives you money, we still have to pay a mortgage, but about 25 banks had said no!

Now we have our college, a building dedicated to teaching and treating people with kinesiology - it's easy to arrive from downtown Barcelona. We also have some rooms for people to stay, if they need to come from a long way for treatment. Our teaching is now certified and accredited, so we can offer continuous professional development courses for teachers, nurses and physiotherapists.

For me kinesiology is amazing! I can particularly talk about postural and muscular skeletal problems because of my background as a physiotherapist. I say to physiotherapists: if you get involved with kinesiology, you will do things in a third of the time it would have taken if you'd used classical physiotherapy.

Francesca worked on a girl aged 21. She'd had an aneurism on the brain and had been put into an induced coma. Her family came to us because we lived in the same village. Francesca went to the hospital and the doctors allowed her to work on their patient through a surrogate (page 18). She came fully out of the coma during a kinesiology session and remembered everything that Francesca had done with her while she was in the coma! She recovered very quickly, and Francesca is still working with her now.

We have a client who had a stroke while on holiday in Canada. It was a disaster for the family - he had to be brought back to Spain in a medical jet and taken to hospital. Once we started working on him, again in hospital, he started to recover faster. He had the stroke four years ago now. As we keep working with him with kinesiology, he keeps on getting back function. Eight months after he had the stroke he couldn't really speak; the doctors said that this is how it would be now and in the future. But neurology is a little more plastic, kinesiology helps to optimize this plasticity, but it wouldn't be easy. Now he's able to walk alone, to be independent; he's gone back to his business. He wants to dance again with his wife. He's not at 100% but he keeps getting back function every month. We have a good relationship with the physios and it's clear that these improvements are definitely linked with the kinesiology sessions.

I could keep on talking - I'm Mediterranean and we talk a lot, but I think this is enough!

Juan Carlos Monge, Montmelo, Spain
www.vidakine.com

Kinesiology: An Application for Professionals

Kinesiology: An Application for Professionals (KAAP) was developed by Christine Ammann of Australia. It was originally designed for nurses and health professionals, although now many other professionals and lay people attend this course. KAAP combines muscle monitoring together with 24 correction techniques and a swift balance procedure to 'unscramble' the body and brain. KAAP is required as a pre-requisite to attend the more advanced Dynamic Kinesiology.

www.dynamickinesiology.com/Kaap.html

KAAP: Christine Ammann, Australia, Case Study

This was a treatment I performed during a presentation demonstrating KAAP techniques to a counseling class of about 30 students.

The client, a lady in her late 50's, presented with a frozen shoulder. She had had this condition for many years and had received lots of different treatments , none of which really helped. With considerable effort she could raise her right arm up to about 40-45 degrees and while doing so she experienced visible pain.

Clearing tests were performed and the only correction that tested up was to rub specific acupressure points on her feet, called gait reflexes. I asked her whether she was willing to take off her shoes so I could rub these points. The class of counseling students looked at me like I was going mad. The question was asked how rubbing her feet could help her shoulder! While rubbing the points I explained the neurological link between the different muscles involved in walking ie legs and arms/shoulders and how rubbing those points can often help to re-establish and balance this electrical circuit. I rubbed the points for about two minutes then asked the lady to raise her arm again.

Previously she had to use tremendous effort to get her arm up to the 40-45 degrees. Subconsciously she put the same amount of effort in to lift her arm, only this time her arm quite literally flung up and over her head – without any pain! The lady was so surprised by this result that she went pale and we had to sit her down and perform an Emotional Stress Release to help her cope with this unexpected positive result!

Two years later, a student who had attended the demonstration came to visit me as a client in clinic. She mentioned that the lady with the frozen shoulder had retained the positive result and still had free movement of her shoulder and arm.

Christine Ammann
South Australia, Australia
www.dynamickinesiology.com.

Neural Organization Technique (NOT)

The Neural Organization Technique (NOT) was developed by Dr Carl A. Ferreri of the USA. He was a chiropractor and also studied Sacro-Occipital Technique, Cranio-Sacral Technique and Applied Kinesiology. NOT teaches that in order to understand our physiological functioning today we need to understand our primitive origins.

NOT gives primacy to the four primal survival systems of the body: feeding, the fight / flight response, the reproductive system and the immune system. These basic systems allowed our ancestors to survive and thrive in spite of the physical challenges of the environment. Other systems of the body are backup systems to the primary survival systems. When any one of the primary survival systems is activated, it takes primacy over all other functions including the other survival systems and any of the other body systems or functions. The activation of these systems is automatic: saliva is produced at the sight of our favourite food, our heart beats faster when we are afraid, etc.

NOT's name comes from the view that the organisation of the central nervous system is central to health, as this system controls and activates the different body systems and functions. NOT practitioners understand that, if the central nervous system is disorganised (through genetics, stress, trauma etc.), this inhibits the true expression of the person's life force and results in dysfunction and disease. NOT seeks to deal with the neurological cause of the problem and not the symptoms.

NOT uses muscle monitoring to find the disorganisations within the survival systems that manifest (through central nervous system activity) as symptoms of some kind. The testament protocols are designed to reorganise the neurological reflex functions and restore the integrity of the primary survival system.

Speaking in 1997 at the Annual International Kinesiology Conference in London, Carl said:

> Once the animal survival systems are intact so the body becomes totally functional, once we become secure in our physical being and are no longer defenceless in the physical sense, we will be able to function on a higher level emotionally. ... We can now deal with the real emotional problems and not a bunch of static. NOT has very specific emotional protocols which work in both the conscious and subconscious levels.

Dr Ferreri died in 2007.

Neural Organization Technique International Inc
www.neuralorg.com

NeuroEnergetic Kinesiology

NeuroEnergetic Kinesiology was developed by Hugo Tobar and originally called Neural Systems Kinesiology. Hugo has a rich and varied background including studying civil engineering in Ecuador and Australia, and living in India for three years experiencing Eastern philosophies.

NeuroEnergetic Kinesiology works with the interplay between metaphysical elements (e.g. chakras and meridians), the emotions, and anatomy and physiology to bring about healing. NeuroEnergetic Kinesiology teaches that every psychological imbalance has a corresponding physical imbalance. It does not matter if the psychological imbalance is a mild, temporary feeling or a full blown mental condition, there will be neurological imbalances that manifest in the neurotransmitters, endocrine system and other parts of the body's anatomy and physiology. At the same time there will also be imbalances within the chakra system and other parts of the energetic anatomy such as the meridians.

The chakra hologram developed by Hugo and Kerrie McFarlane is a central concept in this system. This links the specific chakra imbalance to the subtle body where the imbalance is displayed. The endocrine (hormonal) and nervous systems are seen to be the physical interface of the chakra system. Problems with hormones indicate a chakra imbalance, and vice versa. The chakras have a direct relationship to the nerve plexus thereby directly affecting the muscles and internal organs through the spinal nerves. The practitioner brings the imbalance into the awareness of the client often triggering spontaneous healing to take place. The practitioner may also use tuning forks, acupressure, etc.

As well as the major seven chakras, practitioners also consider 23 minor chakras which are seen to be linked to visual and auditory pathways, internal organ function, joint structure and function, and pregnancy. The nadi hologram gives a protocol for etheric repair. The heavenly hologram works with the five outer-body chakras. This involves issues with grounding, karma and belief systems.

The practitioner uses a combination of acupuncture points and finger modes to access the energetic stress pattern that is at the root of the problem. These combinations are referred to as formats (see page 22). Hugo has added extensively to the list of formats produced by other kinesiologists, including many brain and nervous system formats, primitive reflexes formats, immune and vaccination pathways, biochemical pathways, endocrine system, pathology, physiology, circulatory system, urinary system, structure, consciousness neurology, metaphysical structures, etc.

The practitioners use the framework of the treatment triangle, which is a model that documents the relationship between psychology, subtle anatomy, and physical anatomy and physiology in both healthy states and imbalanced states of health. Using jaw stacking (see page 20), practitioners build up complex stress patterns.

114

The practitioner will trace pathways of stress until the cause is found. There are various recognised pathways, such as neural emotional pathways, auditory & vestibular pathways, biochemical pathways, the immune and vaccination pathways, the developmental pathways, etc. Each pathway has associated formats. For example, structural pathways have formats for muscles, bones, ligaments, tendons, etc. The circulation pathways formats include those for every artery and vein. These allow the practitioner to use muscle monitoring to identify the exact place where the imbalance lies and the cause of that imbalance. Practitioners also work with primitive reflexes (see page 34) and neuro-developmental delay.

Re-balancing procedures include sound, light and acupressure with the exact activity and place on the body being determined by the muscle testing. Meditation and affirmations may also be used.

www.kinstitute.com
www.icnek.com
www.icnek.at
www.acnek.com

Hugo Tobar, Australia, talking about NeuroEnergetic Kinesiology

When I started studying kinesiology in Melbourne, I never thought I would be a developer and travel all over the world teaching it. I would watch my kinesiology teachers and get ideas in my head, but I'd just leave them there.

Just before I graduated I showed Charles Krebs (see page 50) something. He got me to demonstrate it a few times, and then the next day he showed it to all the students and announced that it was a major breakthrough. I thought: well, I have other ideas, so maybe I should start writing them down. I did that and showed them to friends. In 1999 Charles persuaded me to go to the Applied Physiology conference in Arizona. I did a presentation and met lots of people from Europe who wanted me to teach in their countries. I kept on coming up with more ideas, more techniques, and people kept wanting me to teach. I've taught a lot in Germany and now all over the world. I keep doing it and people keep liking it! I fell into it, rather than intending to develop it.

It just seems to grow and grow. In Australia it's registered as a qualified training package – an advanced diploma. Now I'm bringing these qualifications overseas - to the USA, Germany, Ireland and the UK. I think Australia is leading the way in the accreditation of kinesiology into qualifications, but it's got to head this way worldwide - to raise the standards of training and make it into formal qualifications and recognise kinesiology as a valid career.

NeuroEnergetic Kinesiology is based on AP - it's the root it came from; also there are influences from Charles Krebs and the LEAP system. We use formatting (see page 22). A lot of other kinesiologists don't realise how powerful formatting is. Finger modes and reflex points are simple formats, but we use a lot more complex ones. We go into a lot of detail about anatomy and physiology. For example, we've got a workshop just about the immune system. But we also do in depth work with chakras. When I was a student, I was tested and came up as right-brain dominant (see page 33). I was surprised - I trained as a civil engineer and come from a family of engineers - my father, my brother, cousins too. The trainer said that he had observed how creative I was, so he thought that was right, but he also said that my left brain was well integrated. I think that's reflected in NeuroEnergetic Kinesiology. It's important in kinesiology to get the balance right between the two. A lot of the people who are attracted to kinesiology are right brain dominant, so I put everything in flow charts to help them.

Originally I called it Neural Systems Kinesiology to distinguish it from the work I did with Kerrie McFarlane and a couple of others. That was called Energetic Kinesiology, but it's impossible really to separate the work, so I renamed it NeuroEnergetic Kinesiology - I like that name better anyway. Now it's one system - you can't separate it. In fact all the kinesiologies have energetic work in them, even Touch for Health - we learn about meridians there.

When I look back, I'm very satisfied. It has been a real journey for me - personal growth. When I started, I had no training as a teacher - flashes of brilliance between flashes of ordinariness. I was unhappy in my personal life and that made things difficult, but now I'm happy and settled and that has a really positive effect on my teaching. Teaching takes experience and now I've got that too.

I've studied civil engineering, and I studied in India in an ashram; I've even run a T-shirt business. All this is crucial for where I am and what I do now. This is my destiny; doing this is my destiny, for sure. I was put on this planet to do it. All my life has been a preparation for this.

www.kinstitute.com
www.icnek.com

NeuroEnergetic Kinesiology: Tami Davis, USA, Case Study

In October 2006 I saw Jessica (not her real name). She had been sexually abused by her brother when she was around 12 years of age. When Jessica was around 18 years old, she had tried to talk to him before he got married. He had basically told her it was past history and to get over it.

She had suppressed the issues and was now 24 years old, married with two children of her own. She was soon to have a vacation with her brother and mother who lived out of state. She was expecting it to be a very difficult time: her mother had not protected her and had allowed the situation to continue with her brother and did not give him any consequences for his behavior.

Jessica came to me about the vacation; she was almost terrified to deal with her mother and brother. She also had marital issues and had great concern about how her marriage was going. Jessica felt that she did not have a voice in her marriage and that her husband was very jealous, making her feel smothered.

We addressed her inability to be able to be supported about the sexual abuse, and her rage was intense. By using a variety of modalities we were able to discuss and open up her voice. She ended up screaming at her brother and expressing deep rage. The release was incredible: finding the right to speak and express her outrage at what had happened. Telling him in the session that he had no right to take advantage of her - screaming her feelings - the emotions were tremendously powerful. While she was doing this release, I was formatting the brain pathways (see page 22), supporting her when her body jammed using Neural Emotional Pathways and also formatted the throat charka , and using many other modalities to support her in her expression. She left the session drained but incredibly relieved.

She contacted me a few days before she was supposed to be with her family and reported the following: her brother had actually called their mother in deep concern about what had happened with Jessica when she was 12 years old, and said that he wanted to figure out a resolution to the situation. He wasn't even sure himself why it came up at this point, but he felt compelled to address the previously suppressed issue. This was actually two days after Jessica's session with me.

Jessica then got validation from her mother and a very apologetic brother. This began the process of healing the many old wounds between them. Jessica was incredibly amazed and very grateful for the voice that she had been able to have; she now felt supported and heard by her family.

The relief she received totally changed her relationship with her brother, and benefitted her relationship with her mother. The issues with her mother and brother overlapped many of the issues in her marriage, so this also helped her marriage.

Then in March 2007 Jessica came back to do more processing: she wanted to get pregnant. She had one son but was unable to conceive again.

During our session we worked more with her emotional aspects, finding that part of her did not actually want to get pregnant. She was resentful of her husband's over controlling behavior and jealousy and not sure whether she actually wanted to be married, let alone conceive another child.

By addressing the reversal issues (see page 33) in her body, facing the truth of what was really going on, she was able to come to a place of being more united in what she really wanted. She felt more neutral with the issues in her marriage and felt much calmer about her desires for motherhood; she felt more balanced.

In April 2007 Jessica came back and reported that her husband's behavior had calmed down tremendously; he was not so overbearing and even the jealousy had greatly subsided. She came to this session still wanting to address getting pregnant.

This time we worked more on her physical body and her hormones. There were blocks in her cycle and energy, and stresses that needed to be cleared. As we worked on these blockages, issues that were present in her marriage came to light. As we helped her find answers to these issues, the energy started to clear. We supported her body with an herb from Standard Process called Utrophin. I also recommended raspberry tea which she used.

After the session she reported that her marriage was stronger and that she felt much calmer. She was actually enjoying being married and was able to conceive later, giving birth to a second son.

There have been numerous success stories with this work. If the body is in stress, sabotages & reversals occur oft times with many physical ailments. Patterns that get locked in (as early as in the womb or handed down through DNA) are often able to be released or transformed, as you work with clients. Sometimes there is one process and then they are able to make the shifts needed. But other times with deep long term issues they need more NeuroEnergetic Kinesiology sessions. Then they find something that once triggered them is no longer an issue, or much less in degree; they find they have a choice whether they want to react or not. Then the time frame between issues is much longer and the duration of the issue is much shorter. Gradually the client is able to move past the issues that once plagued them so fully.

It is amazing and exciting work in which my life has been forever changed. I have a much greater quality of life; I love being able to assist others to find their own answers to a more healthy and full life.

Tami Davis, West Jordan, Utah, USA
www.tamidavis.blogspot.com

NeuroEnergetic Kinesiology: Annette Reilly, Ireland, Case Study

I was approached in early September this year by a student of mine. She was the grandmother of a little baby boy and spoke to me of her concern about her grandchild, a little baby aged just 3 months old. She told me about how the baby was consistently getting up mouthfuls after feeds and how he seemed to be suffering with a bit of reflux. On the 26th September 2010 I was teaching a workshop called 'Principles of Kinesiology' - by Hugo Tobar, founder of NEK.

The same lady came in that morning for class quite upset and explained how her daughter had phoned her to say she was after finding blood in her baby's nappy when she went to change it. The mother of the child rushed her baby to Cavan General Hospital, where the doctors did a scan only to discover that the baby's bowel had moved up to where his stomach should be. A short time later the grandmother received a second call to say the doctors in Cavan were very concerned and felt they should send the baby to Temple Street Hospital in Dublin to operate. The grandmother was very distraught and asked me if she could surrogate for the baby while I work on her.

With surrogate work a person comes to me for a session and agrees to surrogate for the person with the issue.** Generally I would only do this work for a parent/child relationship, as obviously a parent would not be trying to influence the results for their own benefit, as could possibly be the case with a husband/wife, boyfriend/girlfriend relationship. Her parent or grandparent would only want what is best for the child.

I agreed immediately and I did the balance using my knowledge of NeuroEnergetic Kinesiology. The session lasted approximately 40 minutes, during which time I accessed the anatomy and physiology of the digestive system through the use of a unique formatting system (see page 22) and discovered through muscle testing that the stomach, large intestine and small intestine were all indicating stress. I tested the body to get feedback as to what corrections were needed to balance this stress. I performed the corrections required and continued with defusing the primary emotions of which fear, panic and frustration were all evident. About two hours later the grandmother received another call from her daughter to say that when they arrived in Dublin the doctors did a scan before taking the baby down to operate only to discover the baby's bowel had now moved back into place. The doctors and nurses couldn't believe how it had happened, as they have never seen this issue resolve itself before without the use of surgery!!

This is only one of the many case studies I have come across highlighting the power of this amazing work NeuroEnergetic Kinesiology.

Annette Reilly, Longford, Co. Longford, Ireland
www.neki.ie

** Surrogate work usually involves the client being present. See page 18 for more information on surrogate testing. In this case the baby was not present, and so the work was done distantly. Some kinesiology systems and some kinesiology professional organisations do not recognise distant working in this way as part of kinesiology.

NeuroEnergetic Kinesiology: Ronald Wayman, USA, Case Study

Both of the women had issues with fertility. Both had amenorrhea, meaning they were not having a regular monthly period. In fact, neither had a monthly female cycle that involved a menstruation. One had lost two children due to a liver ailment of the children: one child was still born and the other died two weeks after birth. After that time she was not able to conceive nor have menstrual periods. The other client did not have any pregnancies.

In order to conceive and carry a child full term, it is usually best if the mother has a healthy hormonal response system. If there is erratic hormonal behavior within the body, that could indicate several problems that might cause issues later when pregnant. Thus, it was wise first to consider helping the women with balancing the body so that a regular menstrual period could occur.

With NeuroEnergetic Kinesiology, detailed stresses were found with the ovaries, uterus, hormones, nutrition, emotion, and brain neurology. These stresses were found with patience and with specific formats (see page 22) and modes (see page 21) that powerfully set the stage for releasing these stresses with little effort once they were found. With NeuroEnergetic Kinesiology and with some of the empowerlife emotional balancing (www.empowerlife.com), the calm, stress release options made the sessions powerful and rewarding.

Some of the hormones and the holographic view (see page 31) of those hormones included: progesterone (a particularly important one - it is even named after pro-gestation), estrogen, testosterone, luteinizing hormone, follicle stimulating hormone, gonadotrophin releasing hormone, T3 and T4, adrenaline, noradrenalin, etc.

I found with both women, that there was a tremendous amount of stress with some of these hormones. For example, from the emotional side of things, if there was an issue with an abuser, or a parent, or spouse, the stress levels around progesterone or gonadotropin releasing hormone would increase substantially. Or, if there was a problem with a mineral, the stress level would also go up.

Some of the minerals involved included calcium, magnesium, and potassium, but interestingly, manganese often showed on these women. So I often checked for any related stress. For these women, just taking the supplements was not enough. If there is stress related to a nutritional matter, taking more of it does not always solve the problem. Releasing stress was needed before they could get help.

Both of them had used medical means and alternative means to help them. But not until they received the various stress release techniques from NeuroEnergetic Kinesiology did the other support systems begin to work. It is amazing that particular acupuncture points on the body, held with specific modes (see page 21) with specific procedures for releasing stress can have so much effect on the body.

After several sessions their ability to have a regular menstrual period was realized. Both of them took care of themselves with a good diet, exercise and emotional stability (the emotional processing work we had done helped this a lot).

Both needed to deal with their cycle, the effect of their cycle, fatty acid issues during the different times of their cycle and the other stress levels (nutritionally, physically, and emotionally) that occurred during each phase. Energy kinesiology can take this into account because of how the body memory is stored in the cells.

Now the fertility issues became paramount. There were several considerations, such as, pH levels, follicular cycle issues, polycystic ovarian syndrome issue for one, endometriosis for the other. Candida, fungus, parasites, bacteria, virus were among some of the problems, likewise. With all of these it took some dietary changes and supplementation, but mostly it was the energy release work of emotions using NeuroEnergetic Kinesiology. Taking the time to find the stresses and helping the body release them. Details do matter when solutions are scarce.

Both women needed to consider the ability to carry a child and the health of the child. We considered the important issues of fatty acids and proteins, as well as, other nutritional needs; we looked at the hormonal changes of the mother and child. A mother has a different energy signature when pregnant. Stress on the hormones might be different than when nursing or at other life stages.

Finally, I used the brain hologram work of Hugo Tobar that provided powerful tools for finding any possible connection between fertility and brain neurology. I found several areas of the limbic area of the brain that had great influence. In the hypothalamus, the body reads the blood and determines what is needed. However, if there are problems, communication will be off somewhere. Using the techniques, we were able to find areas of the brain and corresponding neurotransmitters that needed detailed stress release.

All in all, both women have beautiful children today. They both were able to conceive, carry the children full term and they cuddle these cute little girls today, and are very happy.

Ronald Wayman, Utah, USA
www.acnek.com

Neuro Linguistic Kinesiology (NLK)

Neuro Linguistic Kinesiology was developed by Australian Wendy Bennett. NLK is a combination of kinesiology with Neuro Linguistic Programming. It works to increase effective communication, and understanding of the power of language, as well as improve goal setting strategies. It also works with primitive reflexes (see page 34) and uses a range of brain integration exercises. Work is focussed on finding and releasing the blocks which are stopping clients achieving their goals.

Neuro Linguistic Kinesiology: Marion Pawson, New Zealand, Case Study

10 year old young Peter was part of a hockey team. Not that he was good enough, really. The coach would only put him on for half the game. At the end of practice he'd trail in last, well behind the others on their warm down lap around the pitch.

His mother brought him for some Neuro Linguistic Kinesiology sessions. Initially, Peter decided hockey would be easier if he could 'run better'.

I also discovered that he wore special glasses to help him read, spell, and relieve frequent headaches.

Peter's sessions took us to a specific kinesiology protocol designed to improve body co-ordination, provide easy access to his 'left' and 'right' brain, and take the stress out of using his eyes.

When I saw him again there was great excitement! At the end of the very next hockey game his coach had remarked: "Well I don't know what's happened, but you're running!"

At 13, Peter shaped his journey through his teenage years by coming up with the idea of tackling inline hockey! Wherever did that inspiration come from ?! Inline hockey is based on North American ice hockey – fast, furious, and dramatic! And a long way from Peter's current skill levels. Neuro Linguistic Kinesiology became part of supporting Peter's dream, with occasional sessions enabling him to learn the new skills required as he moved up the ranks.

His first challenge was to free up his eye-hand coordination, so he could control the puck skilfully, and at high speed. He was determined, and practiced for hours – skating and manoeuvering the solid little orange disk around a series of obstacles he set out on a flat concrete yard. The pleasure he was getting from his increasing skill kept him at it.

Next issue was developing his peripheral awareness of his team mates. We worked on his recognition of visual and auditory cues so he could pass the puck accurately and 'play team'. I noticed with interest that though rather shy, he took on collecting the team's subs at this point

- interacting socially first, and then graduating to the high-speed interactions on hockey blades that had him setting up passes to his team mates - and scoring goals!

As a young man with a deep voice Peter came for another session at 18. He wanted to be able to anticipate the flow of the game and move astutely in relation to both the opposition and his team mates.

Just before he left home at 21 Peter was awarded the club medal for the Most Improved Adult Player. He had achieved peer recognition of what had initially seemed an almost impossible dream. With the prompting of occasional NLK balances, a shy, not very well co-ordinated boy, became a highly valued and skilful team player, in a fast moving sporting code.

Along the way he also markedly improved his health and social skills. The eyesight skills he developed on the sports field were also in evidence in his reading and spelling. Peter sat papers in the national scholarship exams, which placed him in the top 10 per cent for his year.

Reprinted with permission from *OT Insight* Vol 30 May 2009

Marion Pawson, Wellington, New Zealand
www.mind-body.co.nz

Neuro-Training

Neuro-Training (NT) was developed by Andrew Verity. As well as studying Applied Kinesiology, he has diplomas in naturopathy, homeopathy and iridology. He has also studied the Edward Vincent Jones' personology (the correlation between facial characteristics and psychological traits which Andrew updated and created 'applied personology') and cheirology (the correlations between the physical features of the hands and patterns of consciousness). As a result of this background, NT is a synthesis of these and other modalities and kinesiology.

A central concept is that of the Laws of Natural Recuperation, with recuperation and regeneration (physically, emotionally and mentally) being seen as inherent within our genetic make-up. Another is that of the Model of Universal Principles (MUP) which shows the blocks to our true self-expression and how these result in ill-health and distress. NT grew out of what was originally called Educating Alternatives, which reflects the intention to educate people about the alternatives that are available to them for long-term recuperation and self-expression rather than accepting the alternative of on-going stress and/or the suppression of symptoms. With the integration of more and more Human Science principles NT developed into a system of its own which incorporates kinesiology and many other modalities that have been shown to work.

Tools include hand and face analysis as well as kinesiology. The Neuro-Trainer may use their understanding of facial traits and the relationship between different traits to help clients understand why they think and act in particular ways. Linking facial traits and hand traits with archetypes and enneagrams (personality types) helps clients discover life patterns and enables them to turn these into powerful resources in their lives. The challenges, resources and paths of recuperation are unique for each person. The Neuro-Trainer uses the process of association to add better neurological options to what is already in the life experiences of the client.

The NT basic tools train the nervous system to re-evaluate existing defence mechanisms and become better at adapting to on-going and new situations. Neuro-Trainers believe it is important to find the right context in which to train the nervous system into better recuperation for the long term. Through NT the nervous system is offered more and better options, so that it does not have to react in the same way that it has always reacted, which is often based on fear, habits and inappropriate beliefs.

Drawing on insights from homeopathy and other modalities, NT sees recuperation as an evolving process - from the head down, from the inside out, with symptoms appearing in the reverse order of the original occurrence. This process indicates recuperation rather than suppression of symptoms.

Remedial work includes classic kinesiology procedures and unique NT procedures, as well as techniques and insights from Feng Shui, Chinese medicine, homeopathy, NLP and any other modality leading to recuperation rather than suppression.

The Neuro-Trainer does not work with the standard model of illness and disease but rather focuses on enabling the person to find and experience the resources, insights and options that are needed to bring about profound and lasting health.

www.neuro-training.com

Andrew Verity, Australia, talking about Neuro-Training

I first came across kinesiology when I was aged 17. I'd learnt judo from when I was seven years old, and at 17 I was training to be a black belt. I was part of the Victoria [Australia] state judo team. I was pretty tough. Anyway my father came home one day and got me to hold out my arm and tested a muscle. The muscle wouldn't hold - it blew me right out of the water. He rubbed some points, and then the muscles were even stronger than they'd been before. I knew I needed to learn this. I felt: this is the future and everyone will come to this.

I studied all sorts of alternative medicine modalities as well as kinesiology, and eventually integrated them into kinesiology through various mechanisms. I called the kinesiology system I developed Educating Alternatives. It was a training system. I was attempting to fill in the gaps I saw in kinesiology. I thought there were some common connections between kinesiology and other modalities. I was looking for principles and how all these things could work within kinesiology.

My interest and my integrative research led to more than the definition of kinesiology would allow. I set up Neuro-Training, which allows for a broader concept and even more advanced training. I set up the College of Neuro-Training which is a company in its own right. This is government accredited in Australia and delivers a certificate and diploma in kinesiology and Neuro-Training and eventually, I hope, it will provide PhD training. Neuro-Training also allows us to offer workshops and not just diploma training. It allows me to promote new material for public use. In fact we have 22 workshops that are not strictly kinesiology workshops. They're called Neuro-Activation workshops. They don't involve muscle monitoring. People can combine modules - mix and match - to experience the benefits of kinesiology without learning muscle monitoring. People do get direct benefit, but those who don't get what they need from these workshops go on and take other Neuro-Training courses that teach muscle monitoring.

So we have the College of Neuro-Training for people who want a government recognised formal qualification and Neuro-Training for more advanced training and also for the general public through the workshop format.

The basic format is an open learning system. Students add to what they already know - other kinesiology or other specialist training - it can all be incorporated. We use the amazing value of muscle monitoring to allow people to use the material without getting involved in other people's pre-assumptions.

In Neuro-Training I've incorporated anything that works to make the nervous system function better - based on my own research and, to some extent, on that of others. There's a need for a working model to help the work to be effective. We have an N-T Session Model built from practical, hands-on principles. There's also the Model of Universal Principles. This is more theoretical or philosophical. It looks at relationships - the internal with the external, genetics with behaviour - everything.

People have dysfunctional relationships, not just personal ones, but could be the relationship between the liver and vitamin C, or universal principles and the person's genetics. We're looking at how best to retrain the nervous system to use the resources the person already has, or else to use the nervous system to find the new resources the person needs. We can reorganise and help people to use their nervous systems as genetics intended.

I'm interested in integrating neuroscience with what we do. It's really cool because with the tool of muscle monitoring we can work out what we can do with neuroscience quickly; it takes the neuroscience guys years to figure out what to do with all this new knowledge.

We don't use terms that can be defined as therapy - corrections, cure, diagnosis - they're just not words we use. Our focus is mainly on recuperation - recuperation from a divorce a person had years ago, from a car crash, from an allergy reaction … We don't work on issues; that's too easy and it can reinforce people's bad habits. It's recuperation from issues that gets put into circuit (see page 20). It allows the person to learn neurologically a broader range of adaptations, rather than just a correction for an issue. So we are working at a constitutional level; we're in a much better position to help people with chronic as well as acute problems.

When we work we start by looking for the highest priority context to work in for the person to resolve the problem. I might take 45 minutes of a one hour session to do that. There are many things going on for people, but they're not aware of them till you build a different experience into the nervous system. Our main focus is on the nervous system – it's a training process for the nervous system. It's how the nervous system works with the biochemistry, the unconscious, the neuropeptides, emotions … You have to change how the nervous system wants to operate. For example, if you give supplements, the person may be fine as long as they take the supplements, but you're not really changing anything - they need to take the supplements forever, if the nervous system is not changing its pattern of operation. We find the way it needs to be changed in the context it needs to be changed - that's what we're looking for. Then you're always doing the right thing for that person for their long-term benefit.

We deal first with defences; there are four basic elements to be addressed - physical, mental, emotional and energetic. The mental defence - that's what Freud called the negative ego and we call the negative self. Emotional defences - that are a series of emotional connections that act as a net to fall back into - that can stop people moving forward. Physical defences - we use an adaption from the work of Carl Ferrari (see page 113). Energetic defences - we look at the elemental alarm points in the hara. We resolve these four defence areas so that people don't automatically fall into defences, so that they live life to the full. We help people get out of their stuckness - highly technical term that!

We also look at suppression - so many people have inappropriate life experiences or even therapies that stop them from expressing their true nature. We check for suppression after every new balance.

Once the balance is complete we challenge to see how well the changes will stay in place. If the changes are made and not challenged, it's then too easy for old habits to come back. We use Enoptics which I developed - they're optic fibres with impregnated frequencies.

I've being doing this for 35 years, but I still have what I call future shock with what we can do with this - I'm amazed at what we can teach people to do with this. I'm humbled that we've come so far with our knowledge - but you need muscle monitoring to put it into valuable practice. Now my students - who've studied maybe for two years - can do amazing things helping people, when I've had to study and research all this time to get to this place.

I've never lost interest, because of its ability to amaze me. I'm more excited now than at the beginning. I trained originally as a goldsmith and learnt all these skills, but after 10 years I realised that I couldn't advance anymore; I'd done it all; I'd learnt what there was to learn, so I dropped it. But this work is fulfilling; it's always different; there's always more to learn. Muscle monitoring is an amazing research tool. Sometimes I turn a muscle on and off using spindle cells (see page 38) over and over again – just to see it! I'm amazed at the whole process - it's never-ending amazement.

www.neuro-training.com

Dana Hookins, Australia, talking about Neuro-Training

I was a teacher. I taught mainly Junior Primary but had taught up to Year 7. I also spent some time being a German language teacher as well as a classroom teacher.

I didn't really know much about kinesiology until I started studying it. I had taken our youngest son for some kinesiology when he was about five, because he had been diagnosed dyslexic - through teaching I had heard about it helping with children like him. Our children had always seen a naturopath and so obviously I was looking for something natural to help him. I'd come across muscle testing with our naturopath and so knew that much.

We didn't want him to feel different, and so we all started doing the same exercises (see page 43) as he had to - sort of as an encouragement. We thought we noticed some change but there were other things happening at school as well. Anyway I started doing some of the exercises with my children in the class as well - thought it couldn't hurt.

It wasn't until years later that - long story - but because of things to do with my husband and work, we were moving to San Francisco, so I had to take a year's leave from teaching. Then the company he was going to work for over there went bankrupt. So we stayed in Adelaide, but our children had to be re-settled into new schools, so my husband and I decided I'd continue to stay on leave. I was happy to do so because teaching had been quite stressful near the end - all the bureaucratic stuff you have to deal with.

Anyway I was going to study some natural therapy of some kind in the US and so was looking for the same back here - but it needed to be something that you get a lot done in a year - so just picked kinesiology thinking it was something I could do with the children when back teaching.

127

Back then there was really only one major modality offered here. At the time I had fun studying it - it wasn't a Government accredited course back then.

I got to know some nice people - two are still really good friends. At the end I didn't really know how I'd use it in the classroom and also didn't really feel qualified enough to set up a business. Then I found out about Neuro-Training - which was called Educating Alternatives back then - it was really popular in all the Eastern States and some places overseas.

The author of Neuro-Training is Andrew Verity and what I liked about his work was that his background was naturopathy, homeopathy, applied kinesiology, neuro-linguistic programming - everything he taught had sound reason behind it from his other studies - in my opinion 'not airy fairy stuff'.

So I commuted from Adelaide to Melbourne or Sydney wherever courses were being held - practically on a monthly basis - probably for a year and a half - maybe two - at the same time building up a successful practice here in Adelaide - While I was doing that, I decided that Adelaide needed Neuro-Training back here and so decided I'd train and teach it here. Then requirements changed and it's become part of a Cert IV and Diploma etc.

So I run a successful clinic and am the Adelaide Campus for the College of Neuro-Training Neuro-Training helps people make amazing changes. It's client directed; it's not a step by step process that a person has to fit into - it's a procedure that lets the person's neurology/nervous system direct. Neuro-Training's philosophy is that we have all the innate systems in us - we just might need someone to help facilitate the necessary changes.

The innate systems are the many systems we use internally to achieve the things we want in life - e.g. your nervous system - everyone has one but is everyone training theirs appropriately? Or what about your intelligences - we all have a number of intelligences, and I don't mean just IQ intellect, is everyone using all of their intelligences appropriately in all situations?

Neuro-Training is solution oriented, which means it's helping the person find the solutions that are already there within them - not always focussing on a problem. If we work with problems all the time, all we are doing is letting the neurology know it's ok to have problems - so you 'fix' one 'problem' and then something happens to the person that is slightly different to the 'problem' they just worked on and their neurology goes 'I can't handle this' - and then they have to have that 'fixed'.

Whereas if you're working in a solution oriented way - you are training the neurology/nervous system to look for 'solutions' - so if the next 'issue' is slightly different to the one they just worked on, their neurology goes 'OK sort of the same issue but slightly different that's ok I have the resources to work on that'.

Neuro-Training works in context - finding the influencing context is hugely important - it's the big picture - focussing on a broad theme in a positive way. And checking for Suppression - I wouldn't go to a kinesiologist that doesn't check for suppression - when a person is stopped from expressing they are in fact suppressing.

My clients often ask me if I'm still as amazed at the results from a Neuro-Training with kinesiology session as I was in the beginning, and I say to them: Yes I still get a thrill at how information is uncovered and the right pieces of the puzzle are found and then seeing the changes made by the person, whether that be mentally, emotionally, physically, spiritually.

I remember one of my sons saying years ago when he was quite young: Mum, I think you're lucky because you've got a really interesting job - every person is different with different reasons for coming, so it's not the same day after day. And he is correct - even if you had every client in one day come because of a headache - each one will have a different Context from where that headache came, and the journey of discovering the best path for them to change that pattern will be different.

Dana Hookins, Flagstaff Hill, South Australia, Australia
www.optimum-health.com.au

Optimum Health Balance (OHB)

Optimum Health Balance was developed by Charles Benham, a UK kinesiologists and a TFH instructor, during the 1980's. At a UK Kinesiology conference in 2001 Charles said:

> I didn't start out with the intention of designing a new system, it happened spontaneously out of the way my mind works – and then like Topsy it grew and grew and is still doing so …

Charles originally used body, hand and finger modes (see page 21) in his system, but in 1998 he replaced these with an icon system based on numerical coding. Each icon is a symbol printed on a card. He created a prioritised balancing routine starting with a series of pre-checks to ensure accurate feedback. OHB practitioners take five measurements (physical energy, optimum health level, etc.) at the beginning and end of the balance to monitor change and act as a reference standard.

Then other measurements are made to gather more information, e.g. levels of internal conflict, infection, malignancy, etc., as well as emotional and electromagnetic checks. After treatment all imbalances are rechecked to reinforce the balancing.

The closing sequence of the OHB balance includes checking that the client accepts responsibility for change on all levels and identifying any vulnerabilities to mobile phones and other extraneous stressors.

OHB uses a group muscle test. Normally a practitioner seeks to isolate an individual muscle as far as possible, but in OHB a group muscle test is used to avoid use of a specific meridian indicator muscle as the feedback indicator. The elbow flexor, shoulder or hip abductor group is used and initially checked on both the left and right side of the body. For the gathering of information phase OHB works with the body 'in lock' which practitioners believe forces the body to be honest.

The practitioner uses icons that are designed to have particular energy qualities. These are used in conjunction with muscle testing to determine the imbalances within the body and indicate the areas to be addressed. There is a large range of icons: intermittent problem, denial, dural tension, harmful early life fears, negative mind set, jealousy, female organ, airborne pollutants, cholesterol balance, toxic metal, emotional instability, self-respect, boundary, eye reading stress, temperature control, etc.

There are checks at every step in the balance for, among other things, stress, self-sabotage, hidden agendas, foreign energy and the need to regress to an earlier time when the current pattern was laid down. These issues are important particularly when dealing with chronic problems. Significant concepts in OHB are concealed responses (addictions), reversed responses and compensations. Sometimes the body becomes addicted to something (e.g. drugs, food, allergy and psycho-emotional problems), and the normal response pattern will become distorted. As OHB works with the body "in lock" these problems will show themselves and can be dealt with to ensure the body gives accurate feedback throughout the balancing. In reversed responses the body has become completely "hooked" on one or more of its problems and will resist treatment. Compensations involve unhealthy responses to trauma that often result in further problems or trauma with yet more unhealthy responses.

Charles described OHB treatments as being "based on the use of universal energy converted to bioelectric energy by and through the body of the practitioner or by and through icons devised for the purpose and passed on to the body of the client to enable it to heal itself." (*Optimum Health Balance Part 1*). Usually only one balancing technique is required. It generally involves channelling energy through the hands of the practitioner or through a healing icon. The former may involve the practitioner holding their hands on the client's body or off the body but within the energy field of the client.

There are also icons that can be used for self-healing and to balance the body each day.

www.kinesiologyohb.co.uk

Gill Tarlington, UK, talking about Optimum Health Balance:

Optimum Health Balance (OHB) is very different from other kinesiologies because we work with vibrational icons. When we do that, it appears the body recognizes the vibration of the icons and, using muscle response as feedback, we are having a conversation with the body, with the person's "computer". The system is always leading. Once a practitioner has learnt the basic system, they realise that the system is in control of what happens in the session, rather than the practitioner thinking and deciding what to do.

The icons are used to bring the body into energetic balance, to optimum health on all levels. That's what we are always concerned with, not with symptoms, but with causes and getting the body back into balance.

OHB was developed by Charles Benham. It came about because he wanted to measure what he was achieving in a Touch for Health balance. He thought he would be able to do this using the yin yang symbol and a scale from 0 to 100%. His idea was to muscle test against the symbol at the beginning of the session and get a reading on the scale of 0-100 and then check again afterwards to see how much improvement there had been. But he found that as he rotated the yin yang symbol the value on the scale changed. Charles devised a different symbol – a circle with a straight line horizontally across the middle and with the lower half in black. This new symbol gave consistent reading and was the first icon.

By 1998 the system was 10 years old, and there were over 300 finger modes in use. No one, not even Charles, could remember them all. Charles had been experimenting with icons and had created a numerologically-coded bank against which he muscle tested for relevant icons to replace the finger modes. This proved successful and OHB's 10th anniversary was celebrated by the change to this easy-to-use icon system. It's a living system and today we have over 600 icons, all of which have been muscle tested against this bank using a person with the relevant knowledge.

We have 5 categories of icons which deal with imbalances on all levels: physical, emotional, chemical/nutritional and electro-magnetic as well as one's spiritual being. Information is recorded in the body using the first two fingers. We do a lot of pre-checks, which means we deal with addictions (physical and emotional), reversed responses (see page 33) and fight/flight problems, where the body's switches have not reset as they should after a trauma or whatever.

Importantly too we check for any foreign energy, which is an energetic pattern that doesn't belong within our energy field and is having a negative effect. If all these problems aren't dealt with initially, the balancing actually gives energy to the problem.

Our OHB Scan Card is like an index and is permanently monitored to lead the practitioner to the appropriate icons. On the card are the icons for the pre-checks in case the body decides to be evasive during balancing - and bodies are evasive. The OHB and other system icons include Recreating Wholeness (offering development and advancement), and Soul/Cell Communication (about clearing a path from our 'soul' vibration to enable the cells of our body to communicate efficiently to facilitate optimum health on all levels). The index on the right-hand side leads the practitioner to any appropriate protocols.

And finally we come back to the OHB icon which needs to read 100% indicating that the person has reached their optimum health - meaning best possible holistic wellbeing at the time of the balance.

Optimum Health Balance inspires me with its ability to help people. I was lucky enough to learn from the man who evolved this icon system for having a conversation with one's body, which knows all about itself in a way that knowledge alone cannot match. Practicing OHB is a joy and teaching it totally rewarding. Just sharing my understanding of how one's body can help itself is reward indeed.

www.kinesiologyohb.co.uk

Optimum Health Balance: Susanne Lakin, UK, Case Study

I carried out an 'emergency' balance for an art teacher, John, after he had had heart surgery which involved the replacement of one of his valves.

After clearing the blockages to the balance, including energetically correcting for foreign energy (possible from the blood transfusions he had received), I started the balance by 'opening the lock'.

There was no muscle response to the first three icons in the system (internal conflict, primary emotional states, absolute negative), so I went on to identify the primary problem for his being. His muscle indicated that it was in the electromagnetic category, the actual icon being the one labelled menstruation. In OHB, the actual category in which an icon is found is often unexpected. In this case, we might have thought that 'menstruation' would be in the structural, chemical or even emotional categories. However, OHB considers imbalances in a holistic manner suggesting that menstruation has electromagnetic associations.

You can imagine my surprise when John's body revealed 'menstruation' as a primary problem, as he definitely is a man! Convinced that I must have misread his muscle response, I rechecked carefully and found that, yes it really was menstruation. Since no further information was required, I had no choice but to open the relevant programme in his mind/body/spirit system by muscle testing the icon and adding it into his system. This is not unlike working with a computer when we click on an icon to open up a particular programme, for example, one that checks spelling. At that point in the balance, I made the decision not to tell him what his being had identified, as I didn't want to introduce any disbelief in the system (for him or for me)!

The next specific problem that his body showed was not such a surprise. It was in the emotional category and entitled fear. Age regression (see page 39) identified fear from the time when he was in the ambulance being taken as an emergency to hospital. I asked John whether he had been frightened of dying at the time and he replied: "Not at all – I just knew I wouldn't die even though my heart problem was serious."

I then asked him what his fear had been about, and he replied: "Well, I knew I would have to have six months off work and so would have to do my own painting. And I'm frightened of not actually producing anything." At this point, John realised that previously he had subconsciously avoided doing his own paintings by being too busy working as an art teacher. If he was at home for six months he would have no such excuse.

I decided to tell him about the menstruation icon. John's response was: "Well that makes perfect sense – menstruation is all about the creative cycle after all and maybe my cycle needs a kick-start."

The balance was continued until I had priority to treat. In OHB, after clearing any blockages in the pre-checks which make sure that the muscle response is reliable, we do not treat until all the relevant programmes in the mind/body/spirit system have been identified and opened. In John's case I had to sound my Tibetan healing bowl and move some healing icons through his aura.

After the healing John's levels of health were 100%. (In OHB, 5 different measures of health including vital and physical energy and the person's Optimum Health level are read at the beginning and end of the balance. The Optimum Health level which is a measure of the person's overall health at the time, given their particular circumstances, must be 100% at the end of the session.)

After the balance, John said that he felt very peaceful and relaxed at the thought of expressing himself creatively by getting on with his own painting.

Within 4 months, he had painted and reproduced his own Christmas card for each of his students. Previously, none of them had seen any of his finished work. His creative juices were obviously flowing!

Susanne Lakin
Norfolk and Yorkshire, UK

Pathway Balancing

Pathway Balancing Kinesiology (PBK) was developed by Corrina Kennedy. It uses muscle testing with verbal questioning and a set of manuals to assess and prioritise the client's needs. Pathway Balancing views the person from the soul's perspective, seeing their life as a soul's journey, through embodiment, into a unique pathway towards a specific destiny. Any symptoms of disease, distress or poor functioning are viewed as signs that the person has lost their way along their destined path. The PBK manuals are a combination of natural therapeutic techniques, combined with a description of an upward journey through named levels of raised awareness and higher energetic vibration.

www.pathwaybalancing.co.uk

Pathway Balancing: Corrina Kennedy, UK, Case Study

Lucy came for a balance because she had worked herself into exhaustion. Having had a breakdown in the past, she saw all the signs this time and wanted to prevent another one happening. She described herself as a worrier who never felt good enough in her efforts to achieve success. Recently she had made her dream come true and opened a beautiful high-end clothing outlet. Because she was so exhausted, she was on the verge of giving up her business and going back to her old job again. She was depressed at the thought of this but could see no way out.

I began with basic energy balancing using Touch for Health techniques. Then, using the manual called 'Pathway Balancing - The Healing', I carried out some gentle cranial work which released tension in the occipital muscles at the back of the skull. Lucy was talking about feelings of anger that were coming into her mind. She could remember feeling really cold as a child, and no one doing anything about it. I gently placed a warming blanket over her and we were able to move on to the next set of manuals called 'Pathway Balancing - The Journey'.

We started with the first manual called 'Level 1 - The Individual' and began the imaginary walk along her life's path passing numbered gateways along the way until muscle testing indicated that we should stop at Gateway 6 called 'Living Life Joyfully' and use the Coral Aura Soma Pomander (see page 42) to energise Lucy for opening this energy gateway in her life and we were able to move through and travel in the direction of 'Stillness for Expansion'. Muscle testing then showed that we needed to talk about what this might mean for Lucy, and she realised she needed to take a week off and rest. Now that the business was established and she had reliable help to look after it, this was possible. By the end of her session, Lucy felt relaxed and optimistic about a practical way to resolve her problems.

Lucy came for regular monthly sessions, progressing to Level 4 'Heaven on Earth' after three months and Level 5 'The Dreamweaver' after six months. At this stage she had cut her working week by one day, allowing her assistant to take more responsibility. After 18 months of sessions, Lucy met a lovely new man, and they'd started dating. That was over two years ago, and Lucy continues to have regular monthly sessions for personal development and well-being. Her business continues to thrive; she is still very much in love and her health and energy levels are better than she can ever remember.

Corrina Kennedy, Cambridgeshire, UK
www.pathwaybalancing.co.uk

Professional Kinesiology Practice (PKP)

Dr Bruce Dewe and his wife Joan Dewe are founders and leaders of the International College of Professional Kinesiology Practice (ICPKP).

Trained as a medical practitioner, in the 1970's Dr Dewe faced his own life-threatening health challenges, and became interested in Touch for Health, and in 1977 he and his wife became Touch for Health instructors.

Bruce and Joan created 'extra skills' workshops as an adjunct to existing kinesiology knowledge, and were instrumental in helping to establish the International Kinesiology College with its vision of developing a career for professional practitioners of kinesiology. The Professional Kinesiology Practice workshops evolved to become a series of 60 modules taught by ICPKP faculty worldwide. These units meet national guidelines in Australia and New Zealand

Dr Dewe introduced the emotions associated with the five elements system into PKP and increased to over 100 the number of muscles which can be manually tested, by finding additional correction points for the muscles of the hands, feet, pelvic floor, throat and larynx. The Dewes have added dozens of new correction techniques to the PKP texts.

Bruce says that following the PKP protocol is the key factor in a successful outcome for clients, and as part of that practitioners make extensive use of finger modes to find what is needed. Different modes can be used to find what the imbalance is (e.g. fatigue, misperception, frozen muscle, dehydration, etc.) and also what correcting procedures are needed (e.g. flower remedies, focused meditation, exercise, muscle balancing, etc.).

The finger modes are collected together into categories:

- Emotional modes
- Spiritual modes
- Self modes
- Structure/Function modes (see page 152)
- Electrical modes
- Personal ecology modes
- Reactive modes
- Structural modes
- Other modes

Within each category there are many other modes. So, for example, within the structural modes category, there are modes for the temporomandibular joint (TMJ), injury recall, etc.

There are many different modes, each listed in the manual. There is a numbering system that allows the practitioner instantly to know how to produce the mode. Each joint of each finger is numbered twice – once on the top and once on the bottom. The area across the joint is also named a, b or c. There are more than 370 finger modes (see page 21) and about 500 different techniques.

From their base in New Zealand the Dewes have developed the first training programme for professional kinesiologists recognised by national governments (New Zealand and Australia). Susan Eardley, an ICPKP faculty member in the UK, has been awarded a doctorate by Southampton University for her PhD showing the effectiveness of the PKP protocol in the management of chronic low back pain. Denise Gurney (see below), another ICPKP faculty member is also working on a doctorate on PKP.

www.icpkp.com

Denise Gurney, UK, talking about Professional Kinesiology Practice

The underpinning philosophy of PKP is different from the philosophies of medicine and science. PKP is based on a participatory philosophy which means the client is participating fully in their own session – there is no treating of a problem. The client is fully aware at all times of the process that is going on, how they feel about it, and understands the significance of every correction that is used. The client makes the change; the PKP practitioner is present with them on their journey.

Practitioners of PKP do not use muscle testing in any kind of diagnostic way, but use it to assess movement - or limitations in movement - and to detect stress. PKP practitioners tend to use various numbers of muscles in a session. Muscles in different parts of the body may be tested, or a specific muscle balance using muscles related to one area of the body, such as the shoulder or the pelvic floor.

Practitioners always come back to the physical body, because the body shows how the person is able to move. Eleanor Taylor (see page 138) describes PKP as showing "how the person moves through life and how life moves through them." The physical body shows what is happening for that person, but when it comes to the correction techniques PKP uses, those are not necessarily located in the physical body.

PKP is very broad spectrum - the practitioner sometimes uses finger modes (see page 21) to determine what is needed. As a practitioner you don't have a preconceived idea of what you are going to do, the body will tell you. Finger modes are a non-verbal language. You just don't know where a session will go. I like that aspect of it. You don't have a person coming with a throat problem and know how you're going to treat it. There's an open mindedness about it. You might not even appear to work on the throat, but then the throat gets better.

We might use a whole series of techniques - we might have age recession (see page 39) and clear things at all ages, then a lost acupuncture point. Practitioners don't just sit around thinking up new finger modes from an intellectual point of view. Potential new finger modes are researched worldwide to make sure they work for everyone in every country.

PKP places great emphasis on the amount of personal work the practitioner does before they go into practice. The PKP training is long compared with some kinesiologies, because there is a great amount of personal work included for the practitioner. The therapeutic relationship is seen as being key to effective practice. Concepts such as entanglement and entrainment are important. The non-specific effects of the PKP protocol are many, and have a lot to do with the quality of the practitioner.

A PKP balance is a truly co-creative act, undertaken in a spirit of compassion and non-judgement.

Denise Gurney, Cheshire, UK
www.sustainableself.com

Professional Kinesiology Practice: Eleanor Taylor, UK, Case Study

This session was done for a 53 year old woman, Marie, who was due to have a cervical smear test. She was very stressed about this as the last time she had had one it had been extremely painful and uncomfortable, and she had had to tell the nurse to stop the procedure.

Muscle testing established that the goal for the session was:

> My mind and body are relaxed, confident and positive which enables me to have a comfortable, clear, healthy smear test.

The overall emotion was 'too much concern about the issue'. The stress level over the goal was 76%, and the life energy to achieve the goal was 42%.

Using muscle testing, I checked that Marie was willing and able on all levels to give up the need for the problem, was accepting of the positive benefits that would come with achieving the goal, was determined to implement any changes need for this and was 100% protected during the implementation and outworking of the goal.

Following on from this, muscle testing indicated that the first issue to deal with was: 'I let people know when I feel angry'. This showed up as indicating a conflict for Marie: she believed that she could do this and, equally, that she couldn't. We muscled tested to find the best way to clear this and used meridian tapping with eye rotation and statements to do so.

After this I checked to see which systems were showing stress in relation to the goal using both verbal statements and physical tests - gaits (see page 34), shock absorbers, chakras, intercostal muscles, eyes, ears and negative energy field all showed stress in relation to this goal.

Using muscle testing to find the priority correction, we found that her triple warmer meridian was stressed. In Marie's case this was to do with her having gone into survival mode where she could not think clearly. Her body indicated that this was to be cleared using an Aura Soma Quintessence - no. 4 (see page 42), which is for rest and peace in the middle of stress. The next priority mode indicated by muscle testing was the surrogating self mode, where someone is being overly affected by peer pressure. Other issues cleared involved mixed reactivity involving her aura (see page 13) and hypnotic messages playing over and over in her mind.

The goal was then achievable. The systems checked for stress earlier were now clear. The stress was down to 7% and the life energy was 98%.

To support the process Marie went away with a flower essence mixture combining Australian Bush essences and Findhorn essences, the precise composition having been chosen by muscle testing.

Two weeks later Marie went for a smear test, which proved to be exactly as her body had indicated in the goal - comfortable, clear and healthy.

Eleanor Taylor, Edinburgh, Scotland

Professional Kinesiology Practice: (Letters From A Client Of Marney Perna), Australia

First Letter:

Dear Marney

I am writing to thank you for your professional kinesiology care that we have been enjoying and benefiting from since last June (09). I have been experiencing a wonderful vitality as a result of your treatments and am very happy with the tangible results my 3 children have also been experiencing; such as calmer moods and relief from allergy symptoms.

I would like to share significant news regarding my oldest son, Riley, who is 8 ½. As you know he is a very bright child who has surprisingly struggled academically in school. He has previously been diagnosed with cross dominance (right hand/ left eye) and auditory processing problems.

The biggest area of concern academically for Riley has been literacy. He has consistently struggled to read, spell and write legibly despite now being in Grade 4. His weekly spelling test book reveals that week after week he was getting two or three words correct out of ten, was in the lower end of the class for reading groups and was unable to keep up with copying work from the blackboard in any legible fashion.

Riley has had about 5 kinesiology treatments with you to date and the results are remarkable. After the third treatment his attitude took a noticeable improvement and that week he got 10 out of 10 for his spelling test!! Major celebrations!! He is now consistently achieving above 7 every week. His writing has much improved and homework has ceased to be a struggle between us as he is no longer a bundle of frustration and anger. On the contrary, he is absolutely revved!

At a parent teacher interview last week his teacher mentioned that she is noticing improvements in his schoolwork recently.

If tonight is a good indicator, then Riley is off and running with his reading after his most recent treatment with you last Saturday. He asked for a particular book; which is an encyclopedia style children's book. I found it and he made himself comfortable, proceeding to be enthralled by interesting facts which he wanted to read to me. I think you would need to be a parent of a child who has struggled to read for his entire schooling, who has fought against reading the simplest home reader, who has listened to stories with rapture but never picked up a book to read for enjoyment to realize the amazement and joy of this moment. The most amazing part of the experience was the smile on Riley's face as he laughed over the pages and his willingness to just keep turning the pages and reading on....

Pure gold!!

Marney; I am writing this letter both to thank you and to give you such positive feedback. Your work with Riley has, without a doubt, changed his life. I intend on sharing his experience with the significant school community and hope that even this letter could encourage others to give their children the opportunity to succeed through kinesiology balancing.

Sincerely, Heather Bradford

Second Letter:
Hi Marney

Me again!!

Riley did some reading for me tonight again and his attitude and fluency have definitely improved. I told him I was impressed and he said "yeah, it's good there's people in the world that can help us like that. There must have been a time when only one or two people knew it and they passed it one to other people and finally Marney learnt it and other people are still learning it" He's got it figured out and best of all he knows you have made a difference.

Heather

Written by Heather a client of practitioner Marney Perna, Queensland, Australia
www.kinique.com

Progressive Kinesiology

The Progressive Kinesiology Academy was founded in the UK in 2001 by Elizabeth Hughes and Miranda Welton. Elizabeth has now opened the Academy in Australia and Miranda is Principal of the UK Academy.

Progressive Kinesiology brings together different kinesiology techniques and some other concepts, such as the eye zones, Tibetan elements and reactive chakras. It also incorporates some anatomy, physiology and nutrition. PK works to support the whole body (chemical, nutritional, mental, structural and metaphysical) to empower clients to take responsibility for their own lives and actions.

www.progressive-kinesiology.co.uk

Progressive Kinesiology: Miranda Welton, UK, Case Study

Mrs G, aged 43 came to see me because she was suffering with on-going acid indigestion and bowel issues. Other factors included a history of pernicious anaemia, allergy or intolerance to a number of substances including house dust mites, pet hair, various trees and pollens (tested by the hospital), plus lots of stress and grief about the past. She also had on-going back problems and whiplash from an accident. Life now was really good but her health issues seemed to be getting worse.

Over the last 20 years she had been prescribed various allergy relief medication, plus Omeprazole which is used in the treatment of dyspepsia, peptic ulcer disease, and gastro-esophageal reflux disease. She had also been prescribed: Domperidone (increases movement through the digestive system and is used to treat various symptoms of stomach disorders), Pantoprazole (works by reducing the amount of acid produced in the stomach, relieving pain and helping to repair the damage), Ranitidine (reduces the amount of acid in the stomach and is used to treat and prevent ulcers, to treat gastroesophageal reflux disorder and to treat conditions associated with excessive acid secretion), Amitriptyline (acts on nerve cells in the brain so is used to relieve depression and for people who are also anxious and agitated, or who are suffering from disturbances in sleep), and Gaviscon (used to treat heartburn and indigestion). She has also had many invasive investigations to discover the cause of her problems but none had been found.

The Progressive Kinesiology Treatment:

Many of her symptoms indicated a problem with her betaine hydrochloride acid levels, so it made sense to begin by testing both pectoralis major clavicular muscles at the same time. This indicates if a person has enough betaine hydrochloride acid in the stomach. If this test unlocks, then this points to betaine hydrochloric acid levels being too low for the client's body. Testing showed a deficiency of betaine hydrochloride acid by completely unlocking the double muscle test. A deficiency can lead to pernicious anaemia, and Mrs G. had suffered with this for years, especially as a young teenager and when pregnant. As a result she had spent years feeling totally exhausted. Testing showed that a mixed enzyme and betaine hydrochloride acid supplement was a priority for her body to correct this deficiency, one tablet twice a day with a proper meal, not a snack. Because she was suffering from heartburn, she had always been treated by doctors as having too much betaine hydrochloric acid, but too little betaine hydrochloric acid can give the same symptoms. The clues were already there but no one linked them up for over 20 years, resulting in some pretty awful health conditions for her.

We then went on to work with her emotions, dealing with some repressed anger and grief, which were affecting her intestines. The flower remedy Pine (see page 41) was indicated and is supportive of the metal element/large intestine meridian, which helps with guilt, regret and self-reproach. Testing also showed that an excess of aluminium (from cooking pans etc.) was also affecting this area. Aluminium is a toxic metal and gives many physical reactions in the body. Muscle testing showed that the Tibetan Gem Remedy Gold was a priority to help this, rather than the more conventional approach of using a mineral (such as zinc) to remove the aluminium from the body. The Gold was used to heal the aura (see page 13) around the physical body. This remedy also increases self-confidence and reduces tension caused by too much responsibility; it supports the emotions when we have lost a loved one in death or when someone has suffered from a physical injury. Further testing also indicated that, as a child, she may have suffered from parasites which affected her ileo-caecal valve. The ICV is a small circular muscle known as a sphincter muscle. It connects the small intestine to the large intestine, and its job is to prevent unwanted waste from returning into the small intestine. Because this valve wasn't functioning properly, it meant she was suffering from constipation and other on-going toxic bowel problems. The Gold remedy would help 'heal' the tissue memory of this. Currently there was also a weakness when exposed to yeast.

I advised taking the enzyme supplement and Pine Remedy, avoiding foods with yeast (especially white bread) for at least month. To complete the treatment she also required the colour red for her base chakra (see page 08).

Following our session the client had almost two weeks without any symptoms, and then the stress of work/family issues started the acid reflux again. Testing indicated good levels now of betaine hydrochloride acid so she was able to stop taking the enzyme supplement. During this session we found that she was also being affected by repressed grief from the loss of family members and a beloved pet in the past. An aura remedy showed up to support her spinal problems and the after-effects of the whiplash injury. The remedy would also be beneficial for her emotional body. This is where we can hold old emotions which come back as repetitive thoughts and feelings, like a conversation stuck on replay.

Further treatments will be on-going to support her back problems, food intolerances to yeast and fungi and also to help her bowel problems.

Miranda Welton, Essex, UK
www.progressive-kinesiology.co.uk

Spectrum Healing

Spectrum Healing was developed by Jay Cubitt, an experienced UK kinesiologist. Jay is also an engineering science graduate and was a lecturer in Technology and Maths for higher education. Spectrum Healing uses verbal questioning (see page 22) to focus on working with the chakras (see page 08), the subtle energy bodies (see page 08) and the meridians. Other concepts include the Kabbalah Tree of Life, the Enneagram and the Light body. Practitioners use different healing energies through their hands to bring about lasting change.

www.spectrum-healing.co.uk

Spectrum Healing: Jay Cubitt, UK, Case Study

The conscious mind processes about 40 nerve impulses per second while the subconscious sends 40 million nerve impulses per second to the brain. Therefore our subconscious beliefs and patterns, which are formed by our earlier experiences, direct us with little or no conscious control. This is why disease patterns, depression and other problems can be so difficult for someone to overcome. Spectrum Healing can heal these subconscious patterns quickly and easily and rebalance the brain signals that determine our vitality, health and confident enjoyment of life.

David is a young boy who suffered damage during his birth resulting in diplegic cerebral palsy, and subsequently, severe learning disability and epilepsy. David's problems with mobility meant that he could only bear weight and walk stiffly with a walking frame and awkward gait for short distances. His learning difficulties meant that he had complex language difficulties and also that sequencing was a problem – an example was washing his hands. He had to be reminded to wash first and then to dry each time he tried to do it. A behavioural optometrist had said that he would never develop 3D vision and that he had poor reflexes. He also had eczema which worsened when he went swimming.

At around the time David first came to me, he was 7 years old. I have seen David for five half hour consultations, treating him with Spectrum Healing, and allowing plenty of time in between the treatments in order to assess improvement.

At the time of the first treatment David struggled with speech, was frustrated by his lack of communication and was frightened to try to speak. He had learned to say five words: mummy, daddy, yes, no, more. He was learning signing, but this was progressing slowly.

His first treatment focussed on his very traumatic birth and the effect that this had had on him, especially emotionally. His mother says that after coming to see me for the first time, the change in David was remarkable. Shortly afterwards, David started to enjoy trying out words. He loved the words he was discovering and was enjoying experimenting! At first his voice was quiet, but soon he was using his voice for everyone to hear, showing he had lost his fear of trying new sounds. He would sign something and try to say it too. Progress with speech has continued since this treatment.

His second treatment was in the following October and healing was carried out to integrate six of the infant reflexes (see page 34) that had not fully integrated at or soon after birth, as they should have done. The following April his reflexes were tested again by the behavioural optometrist and found to be good.

In the following 3 treatments we continued to work on his 3-D vision, confidence, speech, eczema, his physical mobility and his reaction to swimming pool chemicals. In the following months his eczema cleared and does not now flare up in the pool; he gained 3D vision, as well as further improvements in confidence and speech.

By December last year David's memory for signing was improving. His signing vocabulary was increasing, and he was putting signs together, which reflected his general improvement in sequencing. By March of 2010 David was more confident and vocal in the classroom. His communication is now good, and he likes to chat (using signing, some gestures and words) with people he doesn't know very well, or has only just met. This was something he did not have the confidence to do previously. He knows that he is mostly understood, which adds to his confidence.

In diplegic cerebral palsy deterioration in muscle power and mobility start to occur around the age of 9 years, and surgery is needed to stop tight muscles pulling the hips out of joint, or damaging the knees and feet. David has been helped by physiotherapy, regular botulinum injections to his leg muscles and Spectrum Healing. He is now 11 years old, and so far he has not needed the surgery that would have been normal by this age. He can even co-ordinate walking sticks and soon may not need his walking frame at all. Previously doctors had said that he did not have the sequencing skills to be able to walk with sticks.

Because the other problems were more urgent for David, we had not focussed on the epilepsy in our treatments, although it has been on the general agenda. His epilepsy has not responded well to the drugs he has been given to control it. In fact, it is now getting worse, so we are starting to focus on it in our sessions.

Jay Cubitt, Leicestershire, UK
www.spectrum-healing.co.uk

Sports Kinesiology

Sports Kinesiology is concerned with restoring muscles to their full range of movement, following accident, injury and long-term misuse. Many of the clients tend to be sports and fitness enthusiast and professionals, but people with restricted movement, weak muscles, dysfunctional posture, poor co-ordination and chronic headaches may also be clients. Corrective work may include customised diet plans and nutritional supplements. Clients are usually given detailed exercise routines so that they learn how to move in the correct way.

www.sportskin.net

Kinesiology: Elise Curran (Client of Chris Carter), Australia

I first approached kinesiology as a suggestion from my trainer, Chris, to help start firing specific muscles in my body, as I was over working, and under working muscles in my body. The next time I trained I realised an immediate change. However, this is not the story that took my breath away.

I am a national champion dance competitor and have been for most of my life. Like most dancers and high sporting achievers I get nervous, and struggle with certain moves which constantly need practice and perfection. All of us can sometimes 'choke' or get stage fright. Even after 20 years of dancing, it can happen to the best of us at the worst of times. My prime example occurred with my first competition of the year; I was ready, I was fit and I knew what I was doing. I was ready to take on this challenge head on. However, the minute I stepped out on to that floor, my nerves took over my body and to this day I have no recollection of what happened. I danced and I finished the competition, but it was not to my standard, and I did not place anywhere near what I was capable of. After this I was very disheartened. Stress was creeping upon me as the following weekend was my next competition, which was going to be a much larger scale, even more competitive and even more important. If I blacked out on the practice comp what was going to happen next week? I started thinking the worst. So next day I spoke to Chris again, and asked him to find me a quick solution to calm my nerves – hoping for a magic little pill to take the next week. His response was to do a kinesiology session. As I mentioned earlier this was not my first time to try kinesiology, but this time admittedly I was sceptical, because this was not a time to be mucking around trying to find out what works and what doesn't. I needed something that was a definite cure, as I had my next competition in less than a week. Chris showed he had a lot of faith in this method of madness, and I have developed a lot of trust for Chris over the time I have known him. I knew he understood how important this was to me, so I took the plunge.

 My session seemed pretty normal, I lay down on the table and just relaxed; I had an open mind and trusted Chris knew what he was doing. About five minutes into the session Chris asked me to begin visualising as if I was back at the competition. So I went deep into my thoughts and remembered how I felt right before I went on stage. As soon as I had begun

145

visualising the event, he realised there was something there, something causing me a lot of stress, and this was overcoming my mind and focus during my competitions; this was clearly something deep and emotional. As we went on, Chris did his thing: holding certain points on my body, pushing against my wrist, and then pressure points on my head. During the session once he had worked out what was affecting me, he read me a passage that described me; it was all to do with the heart chakra. Chris also found that I had other stress which was a kind of visual stress, so every time I would look down, it would cause a reaction that made my glutes [bottom/butt muscles] go into an over stressed state, and my quadriceps [thigh muscles] would shut down and move into an under facilitated state. Chris continued the session; after we finished, I was a little bit dizzy and that was all there was to it. I left and went back to work to finish my day.

After I got back to work I looked again at the heart chakra, and what it represented. Within the next few hours I started feeling awful; I was sad and depressed; all the feelings I had when I went through an extremely hard break up only 10 months ago. I started remembering everything from the break up; the things that were said; everything that happened. I felt like I was reliving it like it was yesterday.

That night I went back to see Chris and he noticed I wasn't happy, I explained to him that the way my relationship ended late last year was very awful. I had such low self esteem, absolutely no confidence left in myself, and I was just a mess. At the time I talked it over, let it out, had my cry to supporting friends, but now I realised that the hard times I went through I never overcame; I pushed them to the side trying to pretend I was ok before I was ready. Since then I have kept living and got to a point where I thought I was over it and free to move on with my life. The next day I was still a little on edge, and didn't feel great, but then I went to training and continued my day as normal.

Two days later was my competition; I competed, and did very well: I had a clear mind, I was focused and was happy with the result of 2nd place. The following week I knew I still had issues that I had to deal with so I maintained them in my conscious thoughts. I spoke to a friend who is also a psychologist, and focused on overcoming the negative thoughts and memories. It's now only a week later, and I already feel like an entire weight has been lifted off my shoulders. I brought all those hidden feelings back to the surface, and now I'm stronger and ready to face them head on.

So that is what I have done, and you would not believe the change. I feel. I am so happy; I can say my smile is not fake anymore; my insides feel like they are laughing and dancing; I am truly happy with myself. I even noticed today I am walking different, with more confidence, and I love the person that I am. That is something no one can take away from me, and I am so thankful that Chris was able to dig into these feelings I had packed away deep into the underground and brought them out to play, so that they are able to leave me free to focus on my life in the present and enjoy just being me.

Practitioner: Chris Carter
St Leonards, New South Wales, Australia
www.dchealth.com.au

Stress Indicator Point System (SIPS)

Ian Stubbings of Australia developed The Stress Indicator Point System (SIPS) in 1992 while studying Applied Physiology with Charles Krebs (see page 50). The concept of the Powers of Stress as developed by Richard Utt inspired Ian to create SIPS. He has continued to develop the system since that time.

Although SIPS is based on an electrical model of the body, it offers a holistic approach from the physical to spiritual including models and theories of energetic sciences.

The Sips Law of Stress is based on Ohm's Law. Ohm's law states that the current through a conductor between two points is directly proportional to the potential difference or voltage across the two points, and inversely proportional to the resistance between them. In the SIPS system the blocks (resistance, in Ohm's law) to the flow of energy (amperage/ current) are identified. These blocks are caused by stress and are cleared so that cells can function at their optimal power (voltage) and return to homeostasis. Once this has happened the body has the ability and energy to heal and function normally.

SIPS uses the same basic simple protocol for the entire system. The SIPS point identifies the type and nature of the stress (muscles, tendons, ligaments, vascular & lymphatic limbic systems, limbic emotions, meridian matrix stress, etc.). The Stress Indicator Point is entered into circuit and then the specific amperage and resistance points are determined and pulsed in order to release the blocks to the flow of energy relative to that stress.

The electrical nature of the body does not just relate to the cells, but also relates to chakras (see page 08), auric fields (see page 13), meridians, etc.

Ian Stubbings talking about SIPS

I got into kinesiology because my eldest boy who was eight at the time couldn't read anything. My sister had a friend who had a sister who was working with Charles Krebs (see page 50) and Susan McCrossin (see page 77). She was a psychologist and referred kids to them. She didn't understand what they did but knew they came back different.

Once my son had been helped, I was motivated to do the basic training, and then in about 1991 Charles brought AP (see page 63) to Australia. I did one of the intensive courses and during the second part of the class I started creating finger modes (see page 21) and other things. I presented what I'd found to fellow students. I've got a bit of a creative bent and had ideas about balancing tendons and ligaments. Richard Utt (see page 63) came out to Australia the following March. I couldn't afford to attend all the courses, so I just attended the Brain Physiology course. I was impressed by Richard Utt and how he emphasised the power of stress on the person.

I found a way of correcting a jammed or over-facilitated muscle. I found that a specific acupuncture point - triple heater 18 on the right side – unlocked over-facilitated muscles. I also found that I could use the gall bladder meridian to establish the amount of stress involved. Shortly after that I was attending a Body Mind Spirit show with Charles. I mentioned what I'd found to Charles. He was really interested and also wondered what triple heater 18 on the left side would show up. He had been working with a lady with motor neurone disease for about a year and found it difficult to get facilitation in her lower leg muscles. He found that, when she held triple heater 18 on the left side, her leg muscles got stronger, and then he could use this to add information into circuit (see page 20).

I realised that triple heater 18 related more specifically to muscle function, so that was the first stress indicator point. I also found points for stressed tendons and ligaments. That was the beginning of SIPS.

I realised that the body was trying to rebalance itself and, when it does, these stress energy points become active. The real breakthrough came when I realised I needed to understand more about power. I don't have a scientific background, so I went and learnt about power and electricity. I developed a kinesiological form of Ohm's law!

The stress indicator point tells you the type of stress and how strong an impact it is having on the body (force); this causes a resistance to the healthy flow of energy. Resistance doesn't show up unless you measure it against a flow of energy.

For example, if you had a pain in a joint, it could be muscle, tendon, ligament, emotional stress or lots of other things. You challenge or scan a list of the stress indicator points to find the first stress, and find whether it's over or under. You check for the appropriate amperage and resistance and then you pulse the points. You enter that into circuit and find if there are more stresses. For some problems there can be four or five different stresses. We have SIP points for all sorts of stresses at all levels of our being - primary emotions, electro-magnetic switching, chakras, karmic choice, and others.

Then you do one simple correction to correct it all. In fact pulsing the points is a general correction procedure, but then we do something specific - could be ESR (see page 40) or the 7 Chi Keys (see page 64) or other simple corrections developed within SIPS. For example, we have the meridian matrix stress and correction technique where we identify that system and ask for the points that need stimulating. Most of the corrections involve the hands and energy rather than physical things like tuning forks or supplements. I've nothing against them; it's just not the way I work.

I also developed other things, such as the continuous recording mode. Pause lock takes a snapshot at a particular time, but continuous recording mode captures dynamic flowing information like a DVD would. If someone is telling you their emotional story, you can hold the continuous recording mode, and then it's all captured - you don't have to interrupt the flow by having to stop and put it in pause lock. If someone has a pain when they do something, you can get them to do the action and capture the whole thing.

The courses I teach offer a holistic approach from the physical to spiritual including models and theories of energetic sciences. It's an integrated energetic model using the insights of Barbara Ann Brennan, Robert Becker and others. Each course builds on the previous one.

148

I've taught in Belgium and Germany regularly and recently in Holland and Canada. I haven't taught SIPS in Australia. I'm not very good at promoting myself and SIPS, and I've been busy with a family business and personal things, but now I'm free to concentrate on this.

I never intended to create this - it just happened. Sometimes I think: "why me?" and "what am I doing with it?" I'm like the programmer - I teach people and they take it away and work with it day in and day out and get really good results - a man with severe sleep apnoea, a woman with ulcers on her leg and face waiting for surgery, a child with a brain tumour - people I teach come and tell me about these things and that's the reason I keep doing it.

Ian Stubbings, Melbourne, Australia
sipskinesiology@bigpond.com

Three In One Concepts

Three In One Concepts (also known as One Brain) was developed by Gordon Stokes and Daniel Whiteside in the USA in the late seventies and early eighties.

The name of this kinesiology refers to the integration of the body, mind and spirit, emphasising the holistic nature of its approach to stress and dysfunction. Three In One concepts recognises that behaviour can get stuck because of previous stressful events. If you learn a new skill and it is stressful, then your performance of that skill will always reactivate the old stress hampering present performance. Stress in the past can lead to unresolved emotional issues that result in problems of self-perception, communications and relationships.

Practitioners work with clients to help them defuse the stress so they can make more liberated and more appropriate choices, based on present needs and circumstances rather than past unpleasant events. Stress is seen as interfering with our ability to see what we need to do to best serve our needs and interests.

In Three In One practitioners are known as facilitators, to emphasise that they facilitate the changes that the client wants to make, rather than imposing them on the client or doing things to the client. (Many other kinesiology systems have the same concept without the name change.)

The facilitator seeks through muscle testing to bypass the left brain (logical and controlling) and access the right brain (awareness, emotional understanding).

As with the other kinesiologies Three In One facilitators see success across a whole range of issues and goals, but in particular assist adults and children improve performance in many areas, including those labelled as dyslexic or educationally challenged in some way. Three In One facilitators frequently also work with people who want to overcome pain, release stress, increase their self-confidence, or removing fears about the past, present, and future. However, the facilitators do not work with named symptoms or illnesses, but believe that by working at an emotional level, the emotions associated with symptoms and illnesses can be defused, allowing the body to heal itself.

Mark Ainley (see page 153) summarises what happens in a session like this:

- Discussing the issue and its impact on life in present time.
- Identifying the source of stress using biofeedback muscle testing (which involves gentle pressure on the arms).
- Exploring how the source of stress relates to the issue in present time.
- Releasing the stress through a variety of techniques that your body chooses through muscle testing.
- Infusing positive awareness to replace the negative beliefs.

- Anchoring the new belief on five levels of awareness (physical, mental, emotional, spiritual, external factors).
- Identifying a new choice and self-talk.

There are two concepts that are central to Three In One: the Behavioral Barometer and Structure/Function.

Behavioural Barometer

The Behavioural Barometer is described as a "road-map of behavioral patterns", and is a way of identifying and eliminating emotional blocks. It was developed through muscle testing and not through just thinking about emotions and their role in our lives. It is central to the work of Three in One Concept practitioners but is also used by many other kinesiologists too.

The Barometer has three primary levels of awareness: conscious, subconscious and body. Each level is seen as interacting directly with the other two levels. Each level has two or three major categories, expressed as pairs. So, for example, the conscious level has these three pairs:

- Acceptance – Antagonism
- Willing – Anger
- Interest - Resentment

The first of the pair is the desired state of mind and the second is an emotional state.

For each half of the pair there are a further 4 pairs. So, for example, under 'Willing – Anger' are:

WILLING	ANGER
Receptive - Adequate	Incensed – Furious
Prepared - Answerable	Overwrought – Fuming
Encouraging - Refreshed	Seething – Fiery
Invigorated - Aware	Belligerent – Hysterical

The facilitator always says the left side of the Barometer first, the desired state of mind, and then the emotional state, e.g.

Receptive – Incensed
Adequate - Furious

This means that the desired state of mind is what the facilitator and client hear first; this quickly activates the desire for the new state.

Although it is important to focus on the desired state (on the left side of the Behavioral Barometer), it is also important to accept the emotions associated with the right side of the Barometer. If the emotions of the right side are denied or avoided, the benefits of the desired state represented on the left will not be achieved.

The Behavioral Barometer is used to identify emotions associated with particular events or goals. Clients are not always in the same place on the Barometer - it depends on the issue that

151

is being focussed on. So, for example, for one issue it may be important to look at emotions related to indifference, whereas for another issue emotions associated with resentment may hold the key. The facilitator tests the indicator muscle while saying each level of awareness. The one where the indicator muscle changes is the one that has the most negative emotional charge. The process is repeated to find the relevant major category and then to find the relevant sub-heading. Once the emotions are identified the kinesiologist works to remove, neutralise or defuse them. This may be done by using Emotional Stress Release (page 40), age recession (page 39), creative imagery, flower remedies, etc.

Structure/Function

Structure/Function is another central concept of Three In One and is used in conjunction with the Behavioral Barometer. Structure/Function emphasises how our genetic makeup and structure affect the way we are in the world. Our structure can give vital clues to how we function, what stresses or challenges us and what we excel at. Each individual has a unique Structure/Function.

Our genetic structure inclines us to behave in certain ways, to find certain ways of being comfortable and safe. Most people extrapolate from this to believe that everyone else also prefers to function in the same way and respond to life experiences in an identical pattern. The concept of Structure/Function challenges this and sees each individual as unique with their own genetic code and way of functioning. When we talk about functioning here we are including our abilities, strengths, advantages, purpose and sometimes our talents. S/F is about how we think, take action, how we automatically express (or not), how we feel things and express emotions, how physical we are and how we have developed our current outlook.

The Three In One manual describes it like this:

> The real purpose for knowing Structure/Function is two-fold:
> To know and accept yourself as you really are, not as what you want to believe you are.
> To know and accept the innate behavior of others, without taking that behavior personally.
> (*Under The Code Workshop Manual 3*)

This does not mean we do not have choice. Three In One helps us work with our existing Structure/Function to accept who and what we are, to make new choices and remove stress. It works to allow us to inhabit more of our life possibilities comfortably and graciously. It also encourages us to accept other people without judgement and blame.

Three In One practitioners use people's physical characteristics to understand better the preferred function of clients. There are three basic types (A, B and C), but it is not a simple case of deciding which type you are. It is more subtle than that: for any given trait (e.g. thinking style, emotional tolerance, glandular orientation, etc.) you may be more type A or more type B or more type C, and this can vary depending on the trait. Type A means there are an absence of cells (so less of a given behaviour), type B is in between, and type C means there are more cells expressing that behaviour.

Each of the types within the traits is related to a particular aspect of the Behavioral Barometer. The manuals also indicate typical self-talk for each. Each type needs to move away from an extreme and towards more balanced behaviour. The manuals offer words of advice for a new perspective.

For example, type A's self-talk on the trait of emotional tolerance typically goes something like this:

> "What needs to be done – and how it needs to be done – has to be obvious to everyone."

And the advice includes:

> "Focus on the immediate right-ness of your own behaviour – which is bound to include having more patience and understanding."

Type C's self talk on the same trait might be something like this:

> "…. An easy going attitude comes naturally to me. And I intend the best even though sometimes I don't perform according to other people's time-tables or priorities…"

The words of advice for type C on this trait include:

> "Your basically broad-minded point of view is fine, philosophically.. but [others]see things differently and they may be more right than wrong."

Working with the Behavioral Barometer, using muscle testing, understanding the self-talk they are prone to and listening to the words of advice helps clients to see how their behaviours and attitudes do or do not serve them and to make new and more empowering choices in their lives.

The facilitator can also use this information to manage the session better for the client, by looking at the physical structures which indicate the best way to communicate with that person, so that the session runs smoothly and to the client's best advantage.

www.3in1concepts.net

Three in One Concepts: Mark Ainley, Canada, Case Study

When I was introduced to Federico in Milan, he was very stressed about traveling. He tended to get nervous the night before a trip and over-prepare, going over his lists and checking that everything had been packed in a tense manner. He wanted to be at the train station much earlier than was necessary - well over an hour before departure - and was constantly worrying that 'everything should be ok'. He would sweat, find his heartbeat accelerating, and be fidgety.

We worked on the eve of his departure from Milan to Zurich, and he was already getting nervous. Having been brought up in a very traditional household, the concept of muscle-testing and asking questions that would be answered by the body was certainly very new to him. However, the information that we were finding was so precise that he soon released any doubts he may have had. The Behavioural Barometer words that were revealed through muscle testing described his emotional state perfectly. The corrections that we did began to ease his stress. And when we age recessed - counting back to see what past memory was being triggered in Present Time - we hit on an age where he immediately remembered traveling with his family. On all their vacations, his father would be driving while he was in the back seat, and his father was always tense and speeding; Federico never felt that he had any control, and trips always had an air of stress and anxiety. We proceeded with some body and energy balancing corrections; he created a positive symbol in his mind to replace the stressful memory, and once in Present Time, created the new Choice 'I enjoy traveling'.

What happened the next day was remarkable. Federico got to the train station and felt fine. The train was delayed but he wasn't anxious. He was sitting on the train before it took off, and suddenly thought, 'Oh my God, I forgot to be nervous.' The entire journey proceeded well and he enjoyed it, even though he had to change trains unexpectedly because the one he was on developed mechanical trouble. What was even more remarkable was the return journey, which by most standards didn't go as well. Seeing how he was a young man traveling alone, Federico was singled out by Italian Customs officials, who gave him a hard time and searched him and his bags very thoroughly under the suspicion of him smuggling illicit substances. They harassed him quite a lot, and yet he found himself extremely calm. "It was as though everything that could go wrong to test me did go wrong, and yet I felt calm the whole time. I couldn't believe it," he wrote. "I knew I would get to where I was going, and I felt safe." He did get home - delayed, and yet calm and confident. He has reported that he has noticed a similar calm state on his subsequent trips.

When past concepts (or 'pictures') we've made about 'reality' continue to create patterns of behaviour in Present Time, they can be experienced as stress and limitation. Releasing outmoded beliefs helps us to be more present in a situation and opens us up to more authentic responses. Even when faced with stimuli that used to cause us stress, we might not even be aware that anything is 'wrong': we can simply be with what is. I am grateful for the practice of Three-In-One Concepts "One Brain" system for helping me and my clients be more at ease.

Mark Ainley, Vancouver, Canada
www.markainley.com

Rita Bozi, Canada, talking about Three In One Concepts

Three In One Concepts has many great tools and provides a lot of insights. It is probably best known for the Behavioral Barometer, but marrying Structure/Function with the Behavioral Barometer gives Three In One its uniqueness. Structure/Function (S/F) allows clients to understand the 51 traits that speak to their abilities, their advantages, their purpose, their strengths, their gifts and their lessons. Three In One helps the client to understand themselves deeply through these traits, so that they can bring their best to themselves and to the world, while fulfilling their purpose.

Under stress or when a trait is in denial, we don't always bring our best to a given situation, perhaps because we doubt our own abilities, or someone may have more of a given ability than we do, or someone in the past has commented negatively on our ability (e.g. "I wouldn't be so confident, if I were you.").

Through the work in Three In One we identify traits, find out how to fulfil our traits (purpose), how to use them to our benefit, how to do our Structure/Function in wellness rather than denying it under stress. Structure/Function also allows us to see that other people's structures can be different from ours. This means they may operate in a way that is different from our way. Understanding this assists in personal relating; we can honour someone else's Structure Function as well as our own.

With Structure/Function we can recognize which traits are blocking our success and which traits will support us better with a particular issue or in a particular situation.

What is also unique about Three In One is that at the end of a session the clients makes a new choice – we don't just dig up issues and leave them as is, we defuse the stress on the issue, and then we invite the client to make a new choice about the issue; with this new choice the client engages differently with their issue. We don't just wait and see what happens; we wake up the imagination, renew interest in our lives, give ourselves the freedom to create new options – the client may visualize or role-play how they see their future.

We use Bach Flower Remedies. In Three In One we use text (read out loud) for each of the flower remedies in conjunction with the Behavioral Barometer. We also use Tao Essences, Maui Flower and Jewel essences. Some practitioners may even use other essences or homeopathic remedies depending on their training.

Although there is a lot of talk in Three In One about the brain, we don't just work with the brain; we look at the emotions, the spiritual needs, the physical body and the energy body. In fact we work with five bodies: the mental, the emotional, the physical, the essential (spiritual) and the X-factor body. The X-factor body deals with the unknown and with external situations - it looks at the question of how I trust myself in and with the unknown.

When we work with a client, we test willingness to benefit from the changes and insights. We test for this not just in present time but also in past. We work with generations - previous generations affect who we are and how successful we are in our lives. The issues of our progenitors whisper through our genes. We also test the readiness of the five bodies to integrate the changes. Sometimes one of the body levels may be reluctant to support a change, because of an old held pattern or belief. We look at why that is and what we need to do to correct that. We use the Behavioral Barometer for this to identify the emotions involved and test for an appropriate correction.

In Three In One we work with a client not on a client. We believe the client/facilitator relationship is a partnership and not a hierarchy. We believe that the client is the best authority on their issue and they already have a solution – it is simply obscured because of fear, pain, or fear of more pain.

At the beginning of the session we test: "Do we have permission to proceed gently?" We always want to proceed 'gently' (rather than blast an issue with dynamite), looking to help the client make the changes in a way that supports them and doesn't stress them. We test every step of the way through the session - "Is this the best choice? The best correction?"

Every time I work with someone it's an adventure, each session is unique, however the work is always anchored in Structure/ Function and the Behavioral Barometer.

Rita Bozi, Alberta, Canada
www.brillianthealingsystems.com

Three In One Concepts: Amanda Lee, UK, Case Study

Natalie (not her real name), aged 35, came to see me the first time just out of interest, with little knowledge of what kinesiology was about.

At our first consultation she had a goal of wanting progress in her career and to explore any beliefs and behaviours that could be holding her back. She also told me that she had lower back pain, stress aches in her shoulders and thrush that she had had for years.

I did all the pre-checks to ensure that her muscles were giving me reliable feedback from her body, but once we started getting into the de-fusion she started to block (her muscles refused to give feedback) - the Bach Flower Essence, Elm 'for feeling the responsibility is too great' was indicated.

I then tested using the Behavioural Barometer and identified that she was feeling indifference, hostility and antagonism and that she needed the correction for body polarity, which is to do with feeling wounded. The correction involves holding some points on the head and rubbing some acupuncture points. Then she needed the correction for transverse flow which is to do with outside influences causing stress to the body's energy field. This is corrected by holding points on the head and on the navel for a few minutes while breathing calmly.

Natalie's body then wanted to be aged recessed (see page 39) to age 14. As soon as we got there, Natalie had an out flow of emotion. She was angry and sad; she stamped her feet and cried just like a fourteen year old. I tested using the Barometer to find out what emotions needed to be released, and we got: resentment, offended, grief and guilt, ruined and no choice. I held Natalie in frontal occipital holding (see page 40) to reduce her stress while she told me about the event that had happened when she was 14. Natalie's mother had found and read Natalie's diary referencing the sexual abuse by her uncle that Natalie had suffered for 3 years up to the age of 12. We were able to talk through this traumatic event and access feelings that had been repressed for 21 years. We then used some visualisation techniques to 'change the picture' of her 14 year old self. I then tested to ensure that the painful emotions of 14 year old Natalie had been defused. In the place of these painful emotions we needed to 'infuse' a strong positive state of being. This was achieved by another visualisation of 'loving arms holding, protecting and comforting me '. This image spontaneously popped into Natalie's mind as I was doing frontal occipital holding with her.

Muscle testing indicated that this visualisation was required as home work along with taking the Bach flower remedy Oak for 'success without trying - attainment without effort'.

Natalie felt elated at the end of our session and said: "I've been waiting 21 years to do that!" This feeling continued for days.

When I told Natalie that I was writing this piece, she wrote in reply: ".....there was also relief as well as elation, knowing that this subject could come up, but that it came up in a gentle way and I didn't have to talk about the facts of it, but that I could deal with the emotions."

Initially Natalie continued to see me regularly for about a year, but now comes just when she feels there is some work to do. She says that kinesiology has changed her life enormously. Her thrush has completely cleared up. She feels more in control of her life and feels she has accepted her past and is now more in tune with her emotions. She can talk more openly about her experiences without feeling sick. Her relationship with her children has blossomed and she is embracing and enjoying her sexuality much more.

Amanda Lee, Berkshire, UK
www.YourHealthQuest.co.uk

Diane Piette, UK, writing about Three In One Concepts

There are many different branches of kinesiology working on a broad spectrum of different aspects and applications of holistic healing, but they all have the same core therapeutic technique, which is the testing of different muscles to identify stressors in order to release them using Western techniques as well as Traditional Chinese Medicine.

The beauty about kinesiology is that we can actually communicate directly with the body and get some precise bio-feedback, so it is important to choose the right technique to help with the healing. This entails actually asking the body what it needs to get better instead of imposing any treatment which might not be appropriate and would therefore slow down the recovery to full health.

After reading about different branches of kinesiology, I decided to study the fascinating "Three in One Concepts" created by Gordon Stokes and Daniel Whiteside. This is a specialised area of kinesiology working to defuse the stress and fear resulting from learning difficulties, past traumas and negative experiences. These blockages create imbalances in the subtle energy system and stop us from achieving our goals, what we really want in life, the best for each of us. Three in One Concepts helps us change these negative images into more positive ones and gives us back the CHOICE to get better.

In order to identify the cause - or negative emotional pattern – behind physical symptoms such as irritable bowel syndrome, chronic pain, allergies, skin disorders, asthma and emotional symptoms such as phobias, learning difficulties, attention deficiency and hyperactivity disorder, ME, anxiety, depression, Three in One Concepts uses a chart called "The Behavioral Barometer". This details an impressive range of emotions which the body will recognize through muscle testing to help identify and understand the negative pattern underlying the issue or any form of misperception about past events.

Most symptoms and illnesses are a conscious or unconscious interpretation made regarding a situation or a person. They don't appear randomly on the body. The area affected will give us a good clue about what's going on. For example, the front of the body represents present time. Any pain or problem on the front relates directly to a present situation. The back represents the past. A burning throat represents something we said and regret or something we should say but can't let out. Headaches represent the pressure we put on ourselves, the heart is related to the love we give and receive. A deaf ear? What is it that you don't want to hear anymore? Neck problems? Who has been a pain in the neck in your life? Each part or organ in the body has an emotion or meaning attached to it. We need to look at it closely and it will help us understand and resolve the issue behind the symptoms.

Because physical imbalances are the result of past traumas or negative experiences, working on these symptoms in present time will not prevent the stressor from reappearing in identical future situations. Therefore, with Three in One Concepts, we can go back in time using a process called "age recession" and identify the CAUSE of the problem itself. For example, when someone has a phobia about flying, no matter how much work they do on themselves every time they fly, like breathing exercises or visualisation, this fear will keep on reoccurring every time they fly. Or dealing with dyslexia in present time and ignoring that the cause of it lies in the past will mean a very slow and laborious process to full learning potential. Children with learning difficulties have to act fast or the system will marginalise them in special classes with no opportunities to get back on the normal program.

Using age recession combined with the Barometer will take us to the very specific time where it all started. The stressor will then be defused with gentle non-invasive techniques such as acupressure, sounds, colours, chakras, meridian therapy, flower essences, emotional energy balancing, visualisation to mention just a few. People will finally find themselves able to deal with problem situations without the same stress reaction.

> Once we relieve the pain, most often the physical symptoms ease off, then vanish.
> When the past defuses from the present, positive changes DO take place.
> Gordon Stokes

As an example, I once worked on someone who had a phobia about closed spaces when in cars. She would become very panicky if the traffic were to slow down in a tunnel or experience sweating, difficult breathing and very fast heart beat in the car bay of a ferry, waiting for the doors to open. During the session, we identified the event which was triggering all these symptoms. Fifteen years ago, she had got stuck in a tunnel for an hour because of a car accident. The other drivers didn't switch off their engines for a very long time and rapidly the air turned foggy with exhaust fumes. She could remember the rising panic and the urge to get out of the car and run. Luckily the other passengers of the car managed to stop her. After using the protocol for phobias which includes some meridian tapping, we managed to change the image of the memory itself. All that work was done during the age recession. After defusing the stress caused by that event, the person never experienced panic attacks ever again.

This example shows how traumatic experiences create energy blockages and will be programmed to reappear in similar or even less dramatic circumstances. But some of them are more subtle and less straight forward. When traumas appear during childhood, they can have terrible consequences throughout one's life. In the case of abuse, mental, emotional or physical, emotions such as guilt, fear, anger or resentment will become buried deep inside as the child will not know how to deal with them. Her energy will be disturbed at the deepest level of the unconscious, the Cellular Memory. This is like a foot print in the soul and the whole system will be disturbed. After a few years or even decades of energy imbalances, physical or mental symptoms will appear. IBS, MS, depression, skin disorder, numbness are a direct result of suppressed emotions. Conventional medicine can only attempt to help in treating the symptoms without giving a chance to the soul to heal and there are good chances that the symptoms will reoccur. Traumas and negative experiences do not only happen in childhood. We face them daily in losing a parent or a friend, moving home, car accident, pressure at work, impossible deadlines etc. They all affect us on an emotional level. With 3 in 1 Concepts, we deal with all these emotions on the conscious level, the subconscious level and the body - Cellular Memory - level to help rebalance the energy.

And where do learning difficulties come from? What if you had a parent at home who repeatedly called you "stupid" or said that you will never achieve anything in life! Or during the first years of school, what if the teacher "didn't like you" and was showing it by picking on you, but you had to go back every day in the classroom to learn how to write and read? Under stress our mental capacities and performances diminish. Some blind spots will appear creating more stress. The pressure increases from parents and teachers and we start imagining that maybe we are not good enough, that we will never solve this math problem that this book is way too long etc. By thinking this way, we start creating a Negative Self-Image which creates even more stress and … dyslexia appears. How children perform at school is a direct result of the Self-Image they've created, what they believe to be true about themselves. The 3 in 1 Concepts program for learning difficulties focuses on changing the Negative Self-Image by identifying the person or the experience causing it. With positive change comes the realisation that more is possible. We go about changing our situation by changing the way we FEEL about it.

Three In One Concepts has a unique way to deal with wounded spirits which need immediate attention. To bring harmony to our male/control and female/creative sides, we also need to rebalance our Polarity Energy. The polarities of the body are waves of Essential energy, the life force itself. They are more directly related to the spirit than either Meridian or Chakra Energy. Each part and particle of our physical body is polarized (has a positive and negative within). If any changes occur in the polarities after an important physical or emotional shock, the whole balance will collapse and the oneness between the body and the mind will disintegrate, leaving the door open to accidents, cancer, infection etc.

To preserve a perfect balance between the polarities is crucially important as everything has its opposite - Yin and Yang, solid and hollow, cold and hot, dark and light, moon and sun - and we need to maintain a perfect harmony within ourselves, the world and the Universe in order to grow spiritually and progress towards higher levels of awareness.

Diane Piette, Derbyshire, UK
www.dianepiette.co.uk

Touch for Health Kinesiology

Touch for Health Kinesiology, often referred to simply as Touch for Health, grew out of Applied Kinesiology and made many of the simpler techniques available to the general public. These self-help techniques can be learnt in a series of workshops often taught at the weekend or other convenient times.

There is some information about the origins and history of Touch for Health (TFH) on page 160 onwards.

Touch for Health differs from other kinesiology systems in that its aim is not to train practitioners but to educate and empower everyone with tools they can use to keep themselves, their families and their friends healthy and happy. Nevertheless many practitioners start with Touch for Health to learn the basic system and how to muscle test and then go on to training in other kinesiologies. In fact some kinesiology systems have the basic TFH courses as a requisite to their more specialised and professional training.

People who want to teach TFH officially have to complete various courses and qualifications. In some countries there is also a move to develop a Touch for Health practitioner qualification for therapists who wish to use it more fully.

A central concept of Touch for Health is that if you take a person with an unbalanced system and rebalance it, you will improve that person's sense of wellbeing. You may not know what has caused the stress and imbalance in the first place, but by rebalancing the body the trigger will be corrected at least temporarily and possibly permanently. The aim of TFH is to carry out these balances regularly in order to maintain health and minimise the possibility of disease. There are several different ways in which the balance can be completed.

Fix As You Go/ Balance As You Go

Balance or fix as you go is a system where each of the meridians is tested in turn using a related muscle, and then an appropriate correction procedure is used if necessary, before moving on to testing the next muscle and then fixing that one. The practitioner checks and fixes (if necessary) the stomach meridian and then moves on to the other meridians in the wheel sequence (see below). In this simple way of rebalancing the person's energy system it is assumed that any imbalance is an under energy. Usually the balancing procedure involves only 14 muscles, one for each of the meridians (see page 09).

Balancing Using The Wheel

In Chinese acupuncture theory the meridians are seen as flowing and ebbing. Different meridians are most active at different times of the day or night:

- Stomach: 7am to 9 am
- Spleen: 9 am to 11 am
- Heart: 11 am to 1 pm

- Small Intestine: 1 pm to 3 pm
- Bladder: 3 pm to 5 pm
- Kidney: 5 pm to 7 pm
- Circulation/Sex: 7 pm to 9 pm
- Triple Warmer: 9 pm to 11 pm
- Gall Bladder: 11 pm to 1 am
- Liver: 1 am to 3 am
- Lung: 3 am to 5 am
- Large Intestine: 5 am to 7 am

The central and governing meridians are depicted in the centre of the wheel as they relate to all the meridians and are not seen to have specific peaks and troughs related to the time of day. The wheel is a schematic way of thinking about the meridians and how they flow and ebb at particular times of the day.

Rather than fixing each meridian in turn when the associated muscle tests weak, the practitioner initially tests a meridian associated with each muscle and makes a note of the result. The kinesiologist also checks the alarm points to find over energy.

Once all the muscles have been tested the practitioner can use the wheel to look for a pattern in the over and under energy meridians.

The possible patterns are:

- Fix As You Go
- The Beaver Dam
- Triangles
- Squares
- Midday-Midnight Relationship / Spokes

The Beaver Dam
In this way of working with the wheel, the practitioner uses the concept of under and over energy (see page 19): over energy in one meridian is often followed by under energy in the next two meridians. Working with the first under energy meridian helps draw in over energy from the preceding meridian and send it on to the succeeding meridian. So, for example, if there was over energy in the gall bladder meridian followed by under energy in the liver and lung meridians, the practitioner would rebalance the liver meridian. This type of blockage is known as a beaver dam as it reflects the way a beaver's dam will stop water flowing down a stream. This is using the Shen cycle, also known as the creation cycle.

Triangles
Meridians run in specific directions either up or down the body. Triangles link together meridians that run in the same direction in the same part of the body. For example, lung, circulation/sex and heart meridians all run on the arms from the upper torso to the hand. Again the pattern that is being looked for is one over energy and two under energy. Again the first under-energy after the over energy is stimulated and rebalanced. This is using the Ko or destruction cycle. It is also known as the grandmother-grand daughter relationship.

Squares

The meridians are also linked according to the extremities of the bodies – two yin and two yang meridians run on the feet, and another two yin and two yang meridians run on the hands. When the four foot meridians are linked together in the wheel they appear as a square. The same is true for the four hand meridians.

Midday/Midnight Balance/Spoke

The midday/midnight concept recognises that each meridian is linked to the meridian on the opposite side of the circle. One of the meridians will be at its peak (the midday meridian) when the other is at its lowest point (midnight meridian): when one side has over energy, the other often has under energy.

Rebalancing

Once it has been established which meridian to work with, the practitioner circuit locates (see page 20) to establish which correction procedure to use. Then the muscle is rechecked and all the alarm points (see page 19) are rechecked too.

Often a goal statement will be developed through discussion at the beginning of the session. If the person is muscle tested while saying this at the beginning of the session, the muscle will usually unlock, indicating that the person is stressed by the statement. At the end of the session the goal statement is rechecked and should not weaken. If it does, Emotional Stress Release (see page 40) is used to clear any remaining problems.

www.touch4health.com
www.tfhka.org

Helena Argüelles, UK, writing about Touch for Health

In modern society there is an unprecedented move towards becoming more responsible for our own wellbeing. We research our conditions on the internet; we inform ourselves of possible treatment options; we are fascinated by traditional home remedies; we meditate, go to exercise classes and see therapists. This model of self-responsibility is at the core of Touch for Health. Those using Touch for Health skills do not talk about 'treating' a person, nor do they diagnose or prescribe. The focus is on attaining 'balance' in order to optimise a person's health and wellbeing. In this way vitality is improved, goals are attained and healing and recovery is enhanced.

Do not be fooled in to thinking that this sounds arcane or vague. It is a simple premise. In the 1960s John Thie was a chiropractor and early student of George Goodheart (commonly thought of as the father of Kinesiology). John had a vision - he quickly realised that the techniques he was learning reached far wider than originally thought. He could see that they were so wonderfully effective and yet so simple that they should not be limited to the realm of professionals but should become part of everyone's daily life. With this in mind he put together a synthesis for the ordinary person that didn't depend on participants having any previous training. This synthesis is now taught in over 100 countries and is called Touch for Health.

The educational model that he developed was quite clear. It would provide safe and easy to use tools to assess, to improve posture and to balance subtle energies through dialogue, muscle testing and the so-called 'touch reflexes'. It would integrate a variety of techniques and philosophies, both eastern and western. Most important of all it would empower all who learned Touch for Health to discover self-awareness, self-care and self-responsibility and to share these new skills with others.

The popularity of Touch for Health has been such that, in addition to the educational model it is now the foundation from which most kinesiology practitioners begin their professional kinesiology training. Indeed many practitioners of other disciplines look to Touch for Health to enhance their existing practice and to take it to a different level. By integrating such wide-reaching knowledge Touch for Health sits easily with other therapies and is widely used in clinics of every conceivable type -conventional, complementary and alternative - all over the world.

The Touch for Health Synthesis is taught over 4 levels, each level consisting of 15 hours study. Some people find that simply taking one level is enough for them but most people seem to get 'hooked' and want to take all four levels and even go on to do proficiency level and professional training. However much is undertaken, knowledge of Touch for Health does not fail to make an impression and change people's lives. The physical benefits are often immediately and obviously evident - postural improvements, reduction in pain, increased mobility. These benefits often give the 'wow' factor as they can be so easily seen. But it is important not to underestimate the emotional and/or mental changes. After teaching Touch for Health I frequently receive comments such as:

- "This workshop has totally changed my life."
- "I'm now able to cope with the stresses and strains that inevitably come up and know that I don't have to take them lying down."
- "I feel empowered and ready to tackle anything."
- "I can't believe what a difference it has made to me physically and emotionally."
- "I never thought I would be able to perform in public but thanks to Touch for Health I can!"

What I find most rewarding as a Touch for Health instructor is that over the period of learning students usually develop their own personalities. They are more in touch with their needs, wants, desires and goals. They are able to communicate more freely and understand their own feelings. They consistently achieve optimum performance levels and enjoy a wellness that they haven't felt for a long time, if ever. All are energised and empowered in the knowledge that they are now their own primary care provider.

For me personally Touch for Health is part of my daily routine and everyday life, as well as my professional life. I came to it late in my career. I was already a practitioner and had studied some kinesiology already. But once I found Touch for Health there was no going back. It gave me a real understanding of how to deal with all that life can throw up. My character developed, I gained confidence, physical strength, and an inner peace that I hadn't been able to access before. It has become like an old friend, who accompanies me everywhere I go, and is there to help me overcome any hurdles I may encounter. I use the techniques, as taught by

John Thie and thousands of instructors worldwide in every aspect of my life. If I am tired and can't focus, if I have aches and pains, if I feel ill or down hearted, if I am to have a difficult encounter, if my children hurt themselves, if a friend needs support - the list is endless. I can't imagine life without Touch for Health and all it has given me. I can't imagine how anyone can get through life without the simplicity and beauty that is Touch for Health!

Helena Argüelles, Newnham, Gloucestershire, UK
www.essentialtimeout.com

Helen Bradley, UK, writing about Touch for Health

It was 1988 when I first discovered Touch for Health at a series of Adult Education classes held by Pat Herington in Chichester. As a Speech & Language Therapist I had a background of orthodox medical knowledge but had also always felt the need to explore more about the workings of mind and body, hence earlier 'dabbles' into meditation, yoga, foods for healthy eating, and fitness in general. Despite my initial scepticism, Touch for Health (especially with all Pat's enthusiasm, commitment and constant desire to share her knowledge) began to make sense. She quickly homed in on my long-standing aching neck (following a whiplash injury) and 'miraculously' the pain disappeared. The massage treatment points for upper trapezius and the neck muscles were a revelation, and I realised how easy it was to continue to help myself. Similarly, I played a lot of badminton in those days and often had an aching right arm and shoulder. Muscle balancing revealed problems with the levator scapulae muscle – relieved by hard pressure on the outer edge of shoulder blade. And, so, Touch for Health became a part of my life. To this day I meet up every month with a friend I met at that first course and we share balances, laughter and friendship with each other – yet another spin-off!

That initial course led me to study Touch for Health 2 and 3 but, personally, I still find the basic techniques the most useful, and we do not necessarily need someone else to actually test or balance us to benefit. I have even successfully suggested massage points to rub over the phone to my daughter in Germany, for example when she was unable to turn her head to one side (neck muscles) or when her legs were very stiff after a marathon run (fascia lata massage area down both thighs).

For some years I was a member of the Committee** which gave me another insight into the workings of Touch for Health and, especially, into the devoted energy the committee members put into the smooth running of the Tuesday meetings, workshops, sharing days, publishing Balance Sheet, etc. Many of those speakers and workshop leaders have been inspirational and practical on numerous health related topics. A few talks I have found obscure and bizarre yet still fascinating. Perhaps the highlight was attending a weekend workshop in 1997 led by Dr John Thie - such a charismatic, knowledgeable and caring person. My original green Manual is well thumbed and falling apart but is still treasured complete with his autograph on the front cover. It is also often used as a reference point to check how best to help aches and pains or sudden minor injuries. For instance, a badly twisted ankle recently responded well and surprisingly quickly to rubbing the peroneus neuro-lymphatic points on the navel and pubic bone. Without that treatment I feel sure I would have been limping around for days.

I strongly believe we do all need to become responsible for looking after our own health and fitness wherever possible, especially with the food and drink we put into our bodies and with the type and level of activity we maintain. We cannot expect our doctors to have all the answers. Modern life, unfortunately, encourages us to constantly abuse our bodies with fast food, sugary treats, alcohol, cars to transport us everywhere, TVs to slouch in front of, computer games to amuse our children, etc. etc. But we must take control! Thankfully, Touch for Health is there to help us understand more about ourselves and even used at its simplest level can be life changing. I am very grateful for finding it when I did.

Helen Bradley, Chichester, UK
** The Touch for Health Centre based in Bognor Regis, UK

Touch for Health Kinesiology: Paul, A Client of (Client), UK

I'm a 39 year old male who has suffered from lower back problems and sciatica since 2001. I was very fit and exercised regularly and have run 5 marathons, the last one being in 2008. I was referred to one of the best physiotherapist practices in South West London and saw my physiotherapist weekly for almost 4 years, but with little improvement.

My back pains and sciatica started to affect every day activities, and I could no longer run. Every day events such as coughing, blowing my nose and driving became painful, and the pains started to severely impact my quality of life.

Eventually I was referred in 2008 to Harley Street* to see a well-known back/spine doctor. Following two MRI scans, the specialist advised that my L2/L3 disc was 'bulging' and that I should consider an operation within the year. He was clear that my back would not heal itself and that eventually the operation was unavoidable. The operation was scheduled to take place in November 2008.

This is a serious operation and the thought of it was extremely daunting. I decided to seek alternative therapy as a very last resort in a desperate attempt to avoid the operation.

In June 2008, following a friend's recommendation, I started to see a Touch for Health Kinesiologist. She was very clear that this would take a while and would require co-operation on my part. I was more than willing to work with her to avoid any back operations.

I visited my kinesiologist approximately every five weeks for over an hour, and she worked with me to 'balance' my body. She gave me some dietary advice and advised that I increase my daily consumption of water, which I adhered to as best I could.

I knew nothing about kinesiology prior to my first visit and was somewhat sceptical on how this could heal a serious back issue such as mine. Every time I visited my kinesiologist I could feel a difference and within 6 months the daily pain I had lived with for the past few years was greatly reduced.

I have been seeing my kinesiologist for 2 years now and am so grateful that I agreed to seek alternative therapy. The improvement to my back means I no longer believe that I will need the back operation. My quality of life has vastly improved too. I do limit my physical exercise to swimming and some cycling and no longer run or participate in marathons.

My back is definitely healing and I have total faith in my kinesiologist, who has clearly demonstrated her ability to heal me. I now believe that an operation should be your very, very last resort and that your body is capable of healing itself.

The same kinesiologist has worked wonders with my wife who has had hip and knee problems for over 2 years. She is completely pain free now and we both look forward to healthy and happy life.

Client: Paul, Surrey, UK (Practitioner: Sandy Gannon, Hersham, Surrey, UK)
www.touchforhealthkinesiology.co.uk | www.kinesiologytraining.co.uk
**Harley Street is in central London and is known for its prestigious doctors.

Touch for Health: Tamara Bausman, Canada, Case Study

Ella (not her real name) was in her forties when she came to see me. Her major complaint was severe diarrhea, which she had been experiencing daily for approximately five years. Ella described her symptoms to me. She woke up in the morning and ran to the bathroom with what she described as 'explosive diarrhea'. She would have 5-10 watery bowel movements all within the first half hour of waking. Her system would then calm down enough for her to make the twenty minute drive to work. During that drive she would have to pull over to have a bowel movement on the side of the road at least twice. Fortunately we live in a rural area where she had a modicum of privacy, but she did have to deal with Canadian prairie conditions and weather: during summer months the mosquitoes here are outrageous, and during winter months the temperature is regularly 20-30 degrees below zero Celsius.

She had previously sought help through the medical system and had had two colonoscopies, both of which ruled out any major medical issues, and she was left with a diagnosis of irritable bowel syndrome.

During Ella's first session with me, the first priority imbalance to show up was (not surprisingly) the large intestine system. All three TFH muscles related to this system were out of balance (tensor fascia lata, hamstrings, and quadratus lumborum). We used neurolymphatic reflex points and neurovascular holding points as the corrections. The neurovasculars took quite a while to switch on. All the muscles tested strong after those corrections.

After that first session using TFH she never had to stop on the side of the road again, and her bowel movements were almost normal.

She had a few follow up sessions, in which we delved deeper into her imbalances. What a life changing experience!

Tamara Bausman, Manitou, Manitoba, Canada
www.completehealth.ca

Transformational Kinesiology (TK)

Transformational Kinesiology (TK) has been developed by Grethe Fremming and Rolf Havsboel from Denmark. They have also taken their system to Germany, the USA, Switzerland and Australia.

When one of them became seriously ill, they found that the usual ways of releasing stress or balancing did not work out. In their effort to find a way to balance the energy system, they discovered that in order to balance the physical body, they had to work from the emotional level; if the problem was emotional, they had to work from the mental level; a mental problem had to be worked at from the spiritual level. They realised that 'the higher heals the lower'.

TK is a synthesis of kinesiology, esoteric healing, holistic counseling, creative visualisation and the Teachings of the Ageless Wisdom, described by esoteric teachers, such as Torkom Saraydarian, Alice A. Bailey, Helena Blavatsky and Paramahansa Yogananda.

TK uses kinesiology to identify the hidden blockages in the etheric, emotional and mental parts of our being that prevent us from reaching our goals. The testing and balancing methods are based on work with the subtle structure of the body: the etheric, the emotional, the mental and the spiritual.

Transformational Kinesiology is seen as one of the practical tools individuals can use for consciously and intentionally engaging in the process of spiritual awakening and the understanding of the energy body. TK works to help the person to be true to themselves and to expand their consciousness and realise their soul's path and purpose.

The TK model includes work with:

- The human energetic matrix
- The 7 basic cosmic energies - the 7 Rays and their associated qualities; spiritual laws, etc.
- Understanding of the vital body (the etheric body), the chakras and the auric field
- The human development through the root races, including the psychology of miasms and the development of our sensory perception
- The path of the soul

The practitioner carries out many of the normal kinesiology pre-tests, including checking for dehydration, over-energy, switching, etc. A goal for the session is set through discussion between the client and the practitioner and then confirmed or adjusted through muscle testing.

The goal is then tested further to bring in a heightened consciousness and more soul involvement. How willing the person is to change is tested using a verbal question. The person may not be 100% willing at this point in time, and the practitioner helps the client identify what the stresses and blocks are, but does not fix them at this stage.

167

Then an action is performed and visualisation has to be done to symbolise the completion of the goal. This will vary depending on the goal but could be being inspired and successful at work, dancing for joy, laughing, or any other appropriate action and visualisation.

The client will also visualise the completion of the goal and identify physical symptoms and complaints that are associated with the stress around the goal.

The practitioner uses verbal questioning to check that the person is ready to complete the balance. The amount of prana/life force the person usually has is identified on a scale of 0 to 100 using muscle testing. Once the goal is established the amount of prana involved in the goal itself is checked. After the balancing procedures are completed the amount of prana is again tested and should now be higher.

Through muscle testing the correct TK balance is identified for the goal, and information shared and discussed with the person. The practitioner will explain about inner leadership and the potential to see the situation from the inner soul level as well as the personality level. Core beliefs are tested from both levels to help the person have some insights as to the learning process behind all that happens to us. When the person is satisfied, the balance can be carried out. After the balance the core beliefs will be tested again to anchor the change in consciousness.

The balancing procedure begins by holding the frontal eminences (see page 40) and reminding the client to activate all their body cells, emotions and thoughts for their goal, so as to achieve as deep a balance as possible. A special creative visualisation procedure is the important part of every balancing process allowing the effect to reach the soul level, dissolving blockages and stimulating a sense of gratitude and forgiveness. Homeplay - visualisations, exercises, etc. - may also be tested and recommended to the client.

TK works to enable people to become more fully themselves and to help them on their spiritual journey through life. Grethe and Rolf believe that permanent healing happens only when a change of consciousness takes place.

www.polarisdk.dk

Eva-Maria Willner, Germany, talking about Transformational Kinesiology:

I came across Transformational Kinesiology about 10-12 years ago, but I didn't have time to study it then. I was attracted by the idea of Ageless Wisdom, spirituality and meditation. Meditation had always been important in my life.

I already taught Health Kinesiology, and later, when I had time, I decided I wanted to learn TK. I studied it in Germany and did courses also with the founders of TK, Grethe Fremming and Rolf Havsboelin. Then I started to train as a TK teacher as well, so I went to Denmark to Polaris, their centre in Denmark to do more training.

In TK the goals that are set are from the heart or the soul - they're not just like being good at school or having a new car. I liked that. In TK we look at what the client is complaining about and look at how that can be used; what lessons can be learnt. It's not just a question of balancing it away. We're always looking at things from a higher level - from the higher self to the lower self - it has this detachment.

We often look back into the past looking for a situation that still has such impact that it is stopping the client from moving on. We work with the person's biography; biography work is revealing and soothing - it allows the client to love and make peace with their past. A person's biography or history is important, but TK helps us to be detached and look at things from another perspective, so that we don't take our own biography so seriously any more. TK teaches you to witness yourself more and more, so that you are not acting from the lower self/ego but from your higher self. If we ran our lives from our higher self, we would act totally differently!

I don't use TK with kids and people who've had no experience of a kinesiology balance, although I know other practitioners do. People have to have a level of consciousness and self-responsibility to benefit from TK. There is the concept of karma - I'm the victim. In TK we also use the concept of dharma - I'm the cause and take responsibility. A client might be crying and we don't necessarily console them that much; we get them to step outside their emotions and look at questions such as: Why am I playing the victim? What's stopping me from changing? TK can be harsh; it doesn't pamper people.

In a session there is a lot of talking and guiding the client. It needs a lot from the practitioner. I find that it attracts people who are open to it. Sometimes I have to take people from where they are and explain it to them. But if someone doesn't believe in, say, past lives, that just doesn't come up, and we only find situations from this life. When we do age regression (see page 39), we find out which subtle body (see page 08) is involved. So for example, if it's the mental body, we ask: What beliefs are involved in the situation? If it's the emotional body, we ask: "What are the emotions involved?" I'm often astonished at what comes out and how people suddenly start remembering things.

When I started learning TK, I found the concept of the different bodies in TK very exciting. Many spiritual traditions do not regard some of the lower bodies as being important, but TK says to train all the bodies. I particularly like the importance it gives to the mental body. There are two types of thinking - concrete and abstract. Concrete are facts; people get so involved with those and will fight bitterly over them. Then there's abstract thinking - this is thinking about what is really important. When people access this type of thinking, they make quantum leaps.

One technique we use in TK is working with symbolic situations. So, for example, the person imagines standing inside a yellow triangle or that there is a star above them. When I first started the training, I didn't believe something like this could make a big difference to people. But when the person imagines themselves inside the yellow triangle, it makes it possible to think about other things - they can see themselves doing things they normally can't do - they're in a different space. It gives an imprint to their mind, to the cells, which "shine" through after the sessions, so that from a deep level or from a higher level - from the essence - change is happening.

TK teaches that if you're always busy (with concrete thoughts and emotions) insights from your solar angel can't get through. Everyone has a solar angel - a protective angel who is with you all the time, through many life times, until you are enlightened.

TK is inspiring; it goes deep for the clients.

Eva-Maria Willner, Schenkenzell, Germany
www.meridianum.de

Transformational Kinesiology Gail Anderson, Australia, Case Study

When I first saw Amy (not her real name), she was 35 years old and single. She expressed her lack of confidence, anger issues, feeling 'stuck' in her life and an inability to hold a long term relationship. She had recently met a new man and was afraid of the relationship going the same way as her previous relationships.

Her first goal was: "I am free to enjoy long term relationships".

There were some deep negative beliefs around guilt, blame and punishment. As a child, she was punished for feeling angry; because of her consequent feelings of blame and guilt, she also had a belief that she deserved to be punished.

Just as they had when she was a child, all these issues had had a profound effect on her ability to maintain a deep and meaningful relationship.

TK is based on the teachings of the Ancient Wisdom, and so we looked at the Spiritual Law of Correspondences which says: 'as above, so below, as within, so without', that everything is connected to everything else. Amy was able to see how this related to the difficulties she was experiencing with her external relationship and to what she was experiencing in her internal relationship, especially to that of her 'inner relationship' in meditation.

One of the issues that also concerned Amy was her dislike of dancing, as she had been invited to a ball by the new man in her life and knew that she would be expected to dance. Amy could remember a time when she had loved to dance but had no idea what had changed that.

The balance took us to age 21 and something to do with dancing. Amy then remembered a party where her boyfriend had criticised her dancing ability, and we found she held a belief that 'dancing is embarrassing'. This was easy to clear during the balancing stage, along with her belief that 'people with confidence have problems'. This belief came from the fact that Amy put on a confident front for others, knowing inside she really lacked confidence. As she said: "....I never wanted others to see I was out of control so I put on fronts to convince people (and myself) that everything was OK." At the same time she was not able to see that other people had difficulties too – again in her own words: "...I could never empathise with others as I saw my own problems as far greater than those of anyone else. Most of the time I was far too caught up with 'my' stuff to even realise or see that others had their own stuff going on." Amy was then able to see that having confidence had nothing to do with whether or not she had problems.

A couple of weeks later I spoke with Amy about the ball, and she said she had had the best time ever; she commented that the most amazing thing was that she had repeatedly asked her partner to dance!

During her next session Amy was still in a developing relationship with this man but talked again about being stuck especially in her work life. She had been stuck in the same job for over 20 years but could not bring herself to leave; her job gave her a feeling of being needed. We looked at issues around needing to be needed and her fear of change. Amy left her job a couple of weeks later and manifested a new and exciting job the following week! Her relationship continued to strengthen, and in the second year of their relationship her partner asked her to marry him.

The next time I saw Amy was the following year, and she was expecting their first child and wanted to clear any blocks she had around labour and the birthing process as she was very keen to have a the best birthing experience possible.

The issues involved here were around loss of freedom and loss of control, and again we looked at how the fears around these issues were reflected for her on the inner plane. A couple of months later she gave birth to a beautiful little boy, breast fed successfully and has since given birth to a beautiful daughter.

She still enjoys a fulfilling 'long term relationship' with her partner and continues to grow in her primary 'long term relationship', that with her Self.

Gail Anderson, Sydney, Australia
www.gailanderson.net

Wellness Kinesiology

Wellness Kinesiology was developed by Wayne Topping, a New Zealander now living in the UK. He's a former geology professor, but now concentrates on teaching kinesiology in 22 countries around the world. Wayne became a Touch for Health Instructor in 1977 before going on to develop Wellness Kinesiology.

Wellness Kinesiology has its origins in Touch for Health and Biokinesiology (developed by John Barton). The normal kinesiology pre-tests are carried out at the beginning of the session.

Stress is a central concept for Wellness Kinesiology, and is considered from various standpoints: emotional, nutritional and structural. Emotional stress may reflect past emotional traumas, current anxieties, worries about what the future holds, self-esteem issues, etc. Nutritional stress includes insufficient water, poor dietary choices, nutritional deficiencies, allergies, etc. Structural stress may reflect physical damage, inappropriate exercising, insufficient physical activity, poor posture, shallow breathing, etc.

Clients are shown through muscle testing what is stressing their system and what effects stress has on their system both physiologically and emotionally. Through this, they learn to understand themselves better and see what changes they need to make to be healthier and happier.

Wayne developed muscle tests involving the eight extra meridians (see page 13).

Correction procedures include Emotional Stress Release (see page 40), meridian tapping (see page 39), temporal tapping (see page 39), brain integration techniques (see page 33), neuro-linguistic programming, nutrition and physical corrections (such as neck and shoulder exercises).

Muscle testing may be used to help clients set powerful new goals for their life that can motivate them to a higher level of well-being. Wellness Kinesiology practitioners also work to help people manage their lives better by dealing with issues such as procrastination and poor time management. The practitioner may also offer advice on exercise, nutrition, breathing and relaxation techniques.

Many of the techniques used in Wellness Kinesiology are taught to clients so they can have simple but powerful tools they can use themselves to prevent ill health and actively promote a healthy and happy life.

www.wellnesskinesiology.com

Wayne Topping, USA & UK, talking about Wellness Kinesiology:

Wellness kinesiology has a very positive perspective, focussing on prevention. The client comes in, and the practitioner listens to their story, their symptomology and what's not working for them. We do a lot of work in the emotional area but nutritional work is important too. We also do some structural work. We're particularly interested in helping people with stress.

The session starts with clearing tests and basic muscle testing. I get them to think of something stressful and show them how the indicator muscle switches off. We start out by taking the emotional stress out of some of the things that are going on in their lives and that are disturbing for them. I show them simple stress release techniques they can use themselves. By then they understand the main tools we are using.

We use two main ways to get into the system to find out what's really going on. We can take a TFH type of approach (see page 160) and check out each meridian through its indicator muscle, find the top priority, and then find the muscle and emotion to balance out that meridian. Alternatively we can circuit localise organ reflexes on the client's body. These were discovered by John Barton, the originator of the biokinesiology programme. Again we find the top priority, and then use that to find a specific emotion to balance out the body.

After finding the emotion we will put it aside temporarily, then find the nutrition that is needed to balance the body. Next we will hold or massage reflex points on the body. After doing physical corrections it is time to do some therapeutic work with the emotions. Now we can tap three specific acupuncture points to put the body under more stress to see if we need to do more work. We're looking for a robust correction, so we keep putting the body under stress and correcting it until we can no longer throw the body out of balance. If we found nutrition earlier, we will see if the body still wants the same nutrition in the same amount now that other work has been done.

Then sometimes we'll add in some acupressure points and physical exercises to improve co-ordination and enhance performance. We may also work with stuck emotional states, such as depression, anger, phobias and anxieties. We use the techniques first developed by psychologist, Dr Roger Callahan for addressing phobias. In Wellness Kinesiology I have expanded that methodology to other stuck emotional states and different meridians based on a knowledge of the Chinese five element model (see page 11).

Because we are addressing the imbalances that the client is presenting with, we get to deal with the current problems in their life, plus previous similar situations, and they usually leave with fewer aches, pains, and other symptoms.

www.wellnesskinesiology.com

Katherine, fourteen, came to see me as a result of a phone call from her mum, who knew a little about kinesiology and was desperate to help her daughter. Katherine (not her real name) was in year 10 and doing her GCSE examination syllabus; she was expected to get high marks in all of her subjects. Katherine had shown signs of a severe school phobia during the Christmas holiday and was refusing to return to school, asking to be taken into care if her parents forced her and if they refused threatening suicide. She lived near a motorway bridge and was threatening to jump off it.

On arrival in the clinic she was sullen, refusing to speak and looking very upset. Her mother had explained the situation over the phone to put me in the picture. I explained to Katherine that although her mother had to be present because she was under 18, she was not part of the session unless Katherine wanted her mother to answer for her and anything Katherine said would be fully confidential. After some more encouragement she explained she did not wish to return to school because of very severe peer pressure from so called friends using emotional/verbal blackmail. This caused her to be distracted in the classroom, when she wanted to be left alone to get on with her studies.

I explained muscle testing to Katherine and then continued with various pre-tests, during this process a massive psychological reversal (see page 33) showed up. This took priority in the first session. I worked on it by tapping on the small intestine 3 acupressure points while Katherine repeated the statement: "Even though I feel miserable I unconditionally love, accept and respect myself." After this the reversal showed as corrected giving us a window to work on the causes. Using the Emotional Stress Release holding points on the forehead (see page 40), together with eye rotations and the emotional finger mode (see page 21) or a brain integration technique (see page 33), we worked on statements around Katherine loving, accepting and respecting herself. Muscle testing showed we then needed to use the same techniques for her stress around close family members. Her growth work at home was to continue to work with the Emotional Stress Release holding points on the forehead, together with eye rotations and the emotional finger mode with some of the statements.

In the second session there was no massive psychological reversal present; Katherine still looked very miserable. Katherine said it was more anger than misery, and muscle testing showed that anger was the priority for the session. The alarm points (see page 19) confirmed that the large intestine meridian was the priority and anger was the stuck emotion. At the beginning Katherine said the anger was 9 on a scale of 0-10; after tapping on the meridian it was down to 7. I then worked with the gamut spot, which brought it down to 6; further meridian tapping got it to 4; repeating the eyes closed and humming a tune with the gamut it was at 1. Testing showed that to bring it to 0 Katherine needed integration time and that there was nothing further to do on this. During this process Katherine said she always felt lonely and isolated at school after an incident when she was 4; Katherine then started crying. Her mother said this was the first time she had ever seen her cry since being a baby. Muscle testing confirmed we did not need to work on this and that the tears were a release. Her growth work at home was continuing to tap on the large intestine meridian.

At the third session Katherine looked much better; she even managed a little smile. We discussed how she now felt; she had returned to school two days previously but had had problems with the new English teacher. The head of Art had praised her work, a first from this teacher. I muscle checked for a priority to work with and it was school. We used the Emotional Stress Release holding points, together with eye rotations and the emotional finger mode whilst Katherine talked about English. Then we did the same thing for Biology. Her body then wanted an age regression (see page 39) to the primary school and age 8. At this time Katherine and her mother explained she had had a succession of teachers in the one year. We used age regression whilst working through each teacher at this time until the muscles locked bi-laterally. When we reached age 4, the incident from the previous session came up. This was broken into small pieces and worked on. There was no growth work at home indicated for after this session.

Katherine continued to progress at school; she did extra work in English to improve her grade. She did really well in her GCSE's and is now the proud owner of 3 A*, 5 A and 4 B grades; she is going on to college to study art, French, textiles and economics. A great result for someone who had been school phobic.

Irene Lock, Southampton, Hampshire, England
www.dealwithstress.co.uk

Wholistic Kinesiology

Dr J Dunn, USA, writing about Wholistic Kinesiology

I began my healing journey as many health care practitioners have, by looking for answers to my own health questions. Why was I tired all the time? Why did I hurt all over? Why did I have migraine headaches? All the medical profession could offer me was prescription drugs to cover up the symptoms. I didn't understand this approach; it just didn't make sense to me to cover up symptoms without trying to delve deeper to find the cause. So, I began to pursue alternatives. Changing my diet and taking supplements that I read about in books and magazines offered no help either. It was only when I was introduced to kinesiology that I began to get my life back.

My first visit to the kinesiologist (who was also a chiropractor) was just plain weird. He had my arm in the air, pushing on it and asking me to resist his push, while he poked and prodded on areas of the body. "What a whack job," I thought. But by this time in my healing journey, no one had been able to help me, and this guy's reputation for getting excellent results led to my willingness to give it a try. He went through his routine and, within minutes, not only did he tell me why I was feeling the way I was feeling, but also what to do about it. I decided to follow his instructions to the tee.

A week later, I was convinced that there was something to this strange procedure. My energy was returning, my brain fog was clearing, and my headaches stopped being a daily occurrence. He had my attention. As I began to visit him on a regular basis, my health began to get better and better. All I could think was "amazing". This very weird technique worked wonders where all others had failed. It was hard for me to describe what I was going through to my friends and family, but they all noticed the difference and began to ask me questions.

"You just have to experience it for yourself," was my reply. My friends and family began to visit him. He became lovingly referred to as the "witchdoctor". They made fun of the whole thing, but they all got results. Allergies were disappearing, energy was coming back, aches and pains left, they slept better and many lost weight. They all just generally felt better.

This amazingly simple, yet seemingly mysterious technique made such a profound impression on me that I decided I wanted to learn more and maybe learn how to do it myself. In 1988, I began my study of kinesiology when I signed up for the Touch for Health class. I loved it! I began to practice on family and friends non-stop. I was relentless. I couldn't get enough of it. It was so fascinating and effective and so much fun.

In 1990, I had the good fortune to hear about a kinesiology class in Albuquerque that was being taught by Karta Purkh Singh Khalsa. At this time I was absolutely obsessed with kinesiology, so I decided to go to his introductory lecture the day before his six-month course was to begin. I was hooked! His technique combined all possible healing techniques into one system. I knew I had to take this course, but I had no money at the time. The cost was $1500.

This amount of money seemed virtually impossible to get. I was a single mom and was working at a bookstore for not much more than minimum wage, but I knew that somehow I had to take that class. Remarkably, the very next day, my tax return arrived and I had exactly $1500 in my hand! I knew it was meant to be! It was a sign!

I began to use this new technique and found that my results with clients were remarkable. I was able to detect their underlying health issues, give recommendations on nutrients, lifestyle changes, exercise modifications, and dietary choices and began getting amazing results with all sorts of conditions.

As I began to build a reputation and practice, I realized that I really wanted to know as much as I could about the human body. I began to think about going back to school for a degree. It had been ten years for me since I went to school, but I felt that my motivation and path were clear. I had no choice but to follow my inner voice and destiny.

I began to take a few courses at the local community college in the evenings. Between being a single mother without child support, working full time, practicing on the side and attending classes it was a full, busy life. I finished my prerequisites in 1990 and with a $1000 in my pocket and my eight-year old daughter in tow; I headed to Davenport, Iowa. I began chiropractic school in January of 1991. Little did I know that it would be the hardest thing I have ever done. Finally I graduated in 1995 and moved back home to Albuquerque. I couldn't wait to get back to the desert.

I began to practice with the original doctor who introduced me to kinesiology. It wasn't long before I had a full time practice. I wasn't finished learning though. Hopefully, I never will be. In 1996 I opened my own clinic and began teaching as well. As I began to learn new and different techniques, I realized that I needed to begin my own technique, which is a combination of all the techniques I had learned, coupled with the information I was gathering through private practice. I began developing my own technique and in 2000 began teaching it out of my clinic. I called it Wholistic Kinesiology. I liked the spelling of Holistic with a "W". It was the completeness or "Wholeness" of the technique that seemed to fit.

It has been, and continues to be, a tremendous journey. I learn things daily from the people I work on by using the muscle testing to ask questions of the body. Some of these questions have never been asked before and forge new frontiers into the realm of healthcare and healing. I have never stopped experiencing that feeling of excitement that I felt on that first moment when I knew what my true calling was. It just gets better and better!

There is more to being well than just not being ill. Let's close the gap between illness and wellness.

Dr J Dunn, Albuquerque, USA
www.wholistickinesiology.com

Useful Addresses: Alphabetical

This list does not claim to be comprehensive. The omission of any organisation or association does not

Accademia di Kinesiologia
Via Rutilia 22, 20141 Milano, Italy
Phonel: 02533634
info@accademiadikinesiologia.it
www.accademiadikinesiologia.it

Akademie für Kinesiologie und Heilkunde
Englitzweg 15, D-88147 Achberg / Bodensee, Germany
www.integrative.de

American College of NeuroEnergetic Kinesiology
8817 So. Redwood Rd, #C, West Jordan, Utah 84088, USA
Phone: 801-566-6262 - USA
ron@acnek.com
www.acnek.com

Applied Physiology
3014 E. Michigan Street, Tucson, AZ 85714, USA
Phone: 520 89 3075
iiap@appliedphysiology.com
www.appliedphysiology.com

Association of Specialised Kinesiologists South Africa
www.kinesiologysa.co.za

Association of Systematic Kinesiology (ASK)
104a Sedlescombe Road North, St Leonards on Sea, East Sussex TN37 7EN, UK
Phone: 0845 0200383
admin@systematic-kinesiology.co.uk
www.systematic-kinesiology.co.uk

Association of Systematic Kinesiology In Ireland (ASK Ireland)
Roe Kilmeena, Westport, Co Mayo, Ireland
support@kinesiology.ie
www.kinesiology.ie

Association Suisse pour la Kinésiologie non médicale
Associazione Svizzera della Kinesiologia non medicinale
www.svnmk.ch

Australasian College of Kinesiology Mastery
info@ackm.edu.au
www.ackm.edu.au or www.kinesiology.edu.au

Australian Kinesiology Association Inc.
P.O. Box 233 Kerrimuir, Melbourne, Victoria, 3128, Australia
Phone: 1300 780 381
enquiries@akakinesiology.org.au
www.akakinesiology.org.au

Australian Sports Kinesiology Institute
www.sportskin.net

Berner Institut für Kinesiologie BIK
Seftigenstrasse 41, 3007 Bern, Switzerland
kinesiologie@bik.ch
www.bik.ch

Bio-Energetic Tools & More
Germany
Phone: 07836 957 9911
bio-tools@seminarhaus-krone.com

Canadian Association of Specialized Kinesiology (CanASK)
Box 45071, Vancouver, British Columbia, V3S 2M8, Canada
Phone: 604 669 8481
office@canask.org
www.canask.org

Canadian Kinesiology Bookstore (kinesiology online shop)
483 Glenholme Street, Coquitlam, BC, V3K 5E1 Canada
Phone: 604 936 5463
orders@kinesiologybooks.net
www.kinesiologybooks.net

Centro Integral de Kinesiología Aplicada
Guerrero 94, Col. Del Carmen, Coyoacán, 04100, D. F., México
info@cika.com.mx
www.cika.com.mx

Classical Kinesiology Institute
81, Lancashire Street, Leicester, LE4 7AF, England
Phone: 0116 266 1962
info@classicalkinesiology.co.uk
www.classicalkinesiology.co.uk

Counselling Kinesiology
www.counsellingkinesiology.com.au

Creative Kinesiology
10 Forestry Houses, Bellever, Postbridge, Devon PL20 6TP, UK
Phone: 01822 880264
info@creativekinesiology.org
www.creativekinesiology.org
www.lifetracking.net

Crossinology® Brain Integration Technique
Learning Enhancement Center, 3704 North 26th Street, Boulder, Colorado 80304, USA
Phone: 303 449 1969
lecboulder@aol.com
www.crossinology.com

Dansk Pædagogisk Kinesiologiskole
www.kinesiologiuddannelse.dk

Den Norske Kinesiologforening (The Norwegian Kinesiology Association)
Postboks 195, Mangleru, 0612 Oslo, Norway
Phone: 0954 37 751
sekretar@dnkf.org
www.dnkf.org

Deutsche Ärztegesellschaft für Applied Kinesiology (DÄGAK)
Nederlinger Str. 35, D-80638 München, Germany
Phone: 0 89-1595951
DAEGAKPAKinD@aol.com
www.DAEGAK.de

Deutsche Gesellschaft für Angewandte Kinesiologie, DGAK
Dietenbacherstr. 22, 79199 Kirchzarten, Germany
www.dgak.de

Dynamic Kinesiology Centre
113 Eyre Street, Seaview Downs, South Australia 5049, Australia
Phone: 403 815 622
ammann@dynamickinesiology.com
www.dyanmickinesiology.com

Energy Kinesiology Association — EnKA®
11322 Golf Round Dr, New Port Richey, FL 34654, USA
Phone: 866-365-4336
info@energyk.org
www.energyk.org

Equilibrium (kinesiology online shop)
PO Box 155, Ormond VIC 3205, Australia
Phone: 03 9578 1229
info@kinesiologyshop.com
www.kinesiologyshop.com

Fédération Belge de Kinésiologie
Rue Herman, 14, 1315 Incourt, Belgium
info@kinesiology-belgium.org
www.kinesiology-belgium.org

Federazione di Kinesiologia (Italy)
info@federazionedikinesiologia.org
www.federazionedikinesiologia.org

Finnish Kinesiology Association
Suomen kinesiolgiayhdistys ry Pelimannintie 13 A, 00420 Helsinki, Finland
Phone: 358 9 - 4789 2189, 358 40 - 821 7115
kinesiologiayhdistys@kaapeli.fi
www.kinesiologia.fi

Gabriele Schäfer-Matthies und Klaus Schäfer (Health Kinesiology)
79227 Schallstadt, Germany
Phone 07664 618118
www.kschaefer.de
www.schaefer-matthies.de

Harmony College
575 Anniesland Road, Scotstounhill, Glasgow, G13 1UX, Scotland
Phone: 0141 954 1796
www.harmonykinesiology.com

Harmony Holistics Kinesiology College
Nenagh, Co Tipperary, Ireland
Phone: 086 823 7714
www.harmonyholistics.com
info@harmonyholistics.com

Health Kinesiology Inc
1304 Asphodel Line 2, RR3 Hastings, K0L 1Y0, Canada
Phone: 705 696 3176
hk.office@hk-training.org
www.subtlenergy.com
www.HK-Training.org
www.HK-Practitioners.net
www.hk4health.co.uk

Health Kinesiology (UK)
Phone: 08707 655980
info@hk4health.co.uk
www.hk4health.co.uk

Institut Belge de Kinesiologie, IBK
avenue Paul Nicodème, 26, 1330 Rixensart, Belgium
www.ibk.be

Institut Français de Kinésiologie Appliquée (IFKA)
6 rue Barginet, 38000 Grenoble, France
Phone: 09 88 77 50 90
info@ifka.com
www.ifka.com

Institut für Angewandte Kinesiologie GmbH (IAK)
Eschbachstr. 5, 79199 Kirchzarten bei Freiburg, Germany
Phone 0 76 61 / 98 71 0
info@iak-freiburg.de
www.iak-freiburg.de

Institute Of Bioenergetic Arts & Sciences
USA
adam@kinesiohealth.com
www.kinesiohealth.com/html/Programs/AP/aphome.html

Integrated Healing
info@integratedhealing.co.uk
www.integratedhealing.co.uk

International Association of Specialized Kinesiologists (IASK)
info@iask.org
www.iask.org

International College of Applied Kinesiology (ICAK)
www.icak.com
www.icak.com/college/contact.shtml - for national chapters

International College of NeuroEnergetic Kinesiology
P.O. Box 904, Murwillumbah, NSW 2484, Australia
0 2 6672 7544
info@icnek.com
www.kinstitute.com
www.icnek.com

International College of Professional Kinesiology Practice (ICPKP)
PO Box 25-162, St Heliers, 1130, New Zealand
Phone: 09 574 0077
admin@icpkp.com
www.icpkp.com

The International Kinesiology College
registrar@ikc-info.org
www.ikc-info.org

Internationale Kinesiologie Akademie
Cunostr. 50-52, 60388 Frankfurt am Main, Germany
Phone: 061 09 - 72 39 41
info@kinesiologie-akademie.de
www.kinesiologie-akademie.de

Internationales College für Neuroenergetische Kinesiologie
Franz-Gruber-Straße 8/8, A-5020 Salzburg, Austria
Phone: 0699 8175 9776
info@icnek.at
www.icnek.at

Japan Kinesiology Institute
zenkinesiology@gmail.com

Japan Touch for Health Kinesiology Association
touch4health@kinesiology.jp

Kinergetics
Philip Rafferty, 88 Emu Bay Rd, Deloraine, Tasmania 7304, Australia
Phone: 03 6362 2657
philip.rafferty@gmail.com
www.reset-tmj.com
www.kinergetics.com.au

Kineseedlight
J-plaza 4F, 2-99 Motomachi, Naka-ku, Yokohama, Japan 231-0861
Phone: 045 662 1456
www.kinesiology.co.jp
www.kinesiology-seminar.com

Kinesiologer
Sweden
www.kinesiologer.se

The Kinesiology Academy
Australia
registrar@kinesiologyacademy.com.au
www.kinesiologyacademy.com.au

Kinesiology: An Application for Professionals
113 Eyre Street, Seaview Downs, South Australia 5049, Australia
Phone: 61 403 815 622
ammann@dynamickinesiology.com
www.dyanmickinesiology.com

The Kinesiology Institute
4712 Admiralty Way, Ste.204, Marina Del Rey, CA 90292, USA
Phone: 800 501 4878
www.kinesiologyinstitute.com

Kinesiology Association of New Zealand
www.kanz.co.nz

Kinesiology College of Ireland
1 Rockgrove, Midleton, Co. Cork, Ireland
021 4633421
ger@kinesiologycollege.com
www.kinesiologycollege.com

Kinesiology Federation (UK)
PO Box 28908, Dalkeith, EH22 2YQ, Scotland
0845 260 1094
admin@kinesiologyfederation.co.uk
www.kinesiologyfederation.co.uk

Life-Work Potential Limited (the author's kinesiology online shop)
www.lifeworkpotential.com

Neural Organization Technique International Inc
www.neuralorg.com

Neuro-Training P/L
100 Magellan St, First Floor, Lismore, NSW 2480, Australia
Phone: 02 66221514
info@neuro-training.com
www.neuro-training.com

Optimum Health Balance
23 Church Lane, Burgh-next-Aylsham, Norwich, NR11 6TR, UK
Phone: 01263 732197
gill@kinesiologyohb.co.uk
www.kinesiologyohb.co.uk

Österreichischer Berufsverband für Kinesiologie (ÖBK)
A-1030 Wien, Kegelgasse 40/1, Austria
Phone: 0676 409 19 50
sekretariat@kinesiologie-oebk.at
www.kinesiologie-oebk.at

Polaris International College (Transformational Kinesiology)
Kyndeløse Strandvej 22, DK-4070 Kirke Hyllinge, Denmark
Phone: 46 4066 50
adm@polariscentret.dk
www.polarisdk.dk

Progressive Kinesiology Academy
10 Barn Fields, Stanway, Colchester, Essex, CO3 0WL, UK
Phone: 01206 570143
info@progressive-kinesiology.co.uk
www.progressive-kinesiology.co.uk

Sips Kinesiology Pty Ltd
21 Maroong Drive, Research, Victoria 3095, Australia
Phone: 03 9437 2495
Sipskinesiology@bigpond.com

Svenska Kinesiologiskolan
www.kinesiologi.se

Schweizerischer Verband Nicht-Medizinische Kinesiologie
www.svnmk.ch

Touch for Health Instructors Association of Australia
www.touch4health.org.au
email@touch4health.org.au

Touch for Health Kinesiology Association
7121 New Light Trail, Chapel Hill, NC, 27516, USA
Phone: 919-969-0027
admin@TFHKA.org
www.TFHKA.org

U.S. Kinesiology Training Institute
7121 New Light Trail, Chapel Hill, NC 27516, USA
greentfh@mindspring.com
www.uskinesiology.com

VAK Verlags GmbH (kinesiology online shop)
Eschbachstraße 5, 79199 Kirchzarten, Germany
Phone: 07661-9871-50
info@vakverlag.de
www.vakverlag.de

Vibrana - Schäfer und Matthies GbR (kinesiology online shop)
79227 Schallstadt, Germany
Phone 07664 617277
www.vibrana.de

Vida kinesiologia
c/ onze de setembre 9 -11 passatge, 08160 Montmelo, Spain
Phone: 935684024
vida@vidakine.com
www.vidakine.com

185

Useful Addresses: By Country

Many of the organisations listed under the International heading also have presences in individual countries. Please see their web sites for more information.

International

Please note, telephone numbers are shown as though you are dialling from within the country.

Applied Physiology
3014 E. Michigan Street, Tucson, AZ 85714, USA
Phone: 520 89 3075
iiap@appliedphysiology.com
www.appliedphysiology.com

Health Kinesiology Inc
1304 Asphodel Line 2, RR3 Hastings, K0L 1Y0, Canada
Phone: 705 696 3176
hk.office@hk-training.org
www.subtlenergy.com
www.HK-Training.org
www.HK-Practitioners.net
www.hk4health.co.uk

Integrated Healing
info@integratedhealing.co.uk
www.integratedhealing.co.uk

International Association of Specialized Kinesiologists (IASK)
info@iask.org
www.iask.org

International College of Applied Kinesiology (ICAK)
www.icak.com
www.icak.com/college/contact.shtml - for national chapters

International College of NeuroEnergetic Kinesiology
P.O. Box 904, Murwillumbah, NSW 2484, Australia
0 2 6672 7544
info@icnek.com
www.kinstitute.com
www.icnek.com

International College of Professional Kinesiology Practice (ICPKP)
PO Box 25-162, St Heliers, 1130, New Zealand
Phone: 09 574 0077
admin@icpkp.com
www.icpkp.com

The International Kinesiology College
registrar@ikc-info.org
www.ikc-info.org

Internationales College für Neuroenergetische Kinesiologie
Franz-Gruber-Straße 8/8, A-5020 Salzburg, Austria
Phone: 0699 8175 9776
info@icnek.at
www.icnek.at

Kinergetics
Philip Rafferty, 88 Emu Bay Rd, Deloraine, Tasmania 7304, Australia
Phone: 03 6362 2657
philip.rafferty@gmail.com
www.reset-tmj.com
www.kinergetics.com.au

Life-Work Potential Limited (the author's kinesiology online shop)
www.lifeworkpotential.com

Neuro-Training P/L
100 Magellan St, First Floor, Lismore, NSW 2480, Australia
Phone: 02 66221514
info@neuro-training.com
www.neuro-training.com

Neural Organization Technique International Inc
www.neuralorg.com

Austria

Internationales College für Neuroenergetische Kinesiologie
Franz-Gruber-Straße 8/8, A-5020 Salzburg, Austria
Phone: 0699 8175 9776
info@icnek.at
www.icnek.at

Österreichischer Berufsverband für Kinesiologie (ÖBK)
A-1030 Wien, Kegelgasse 40/1, Austria
Phone: 0676 409 19 50
sekretariat@kinesiologie-oebk.at
www.kinesiologie-oebk.at

Australia

Australasian College of Kinesiology Mastery
info@ackm.edu.au
www.ackm.edu.au or www.kinesiology.edu.au

Australian Kinesiology Association Inc.
P.O. Box 233 Kerrimuir, Melbourne, Victoria, 3128, Australia
Phone: 1300 780 381
enquiries@akakinesiology.org.au
www.akakinesiology.org.au

Australian Sports Kinesiology Institute
www.sportskin.net

Counselling Kinesiology
www.counsellingkinesiology.com.au

Dynamic Kinesiology Centre
113 Eyre Street, Seaview Downs, South Australia 5049, Australia
Phone: 403 815 622
ammann@dynamickinesiology.com
www.dyanmickinesiology.com

Equilibrium (kinesiology online shop)
PO Box 155, Ormond VIC 3205, Australia
Phone: 03 9578 1229
info@kinesiologyshop.com
www.kinesiologyshop.com

International College of NeuroEnergetic Kinesiology
P.O. Box 904, Murwillumbah, NSW 2484, Australia
06672 7544
info@icnek.com
www.kinstitute.com
www.icnek.com

Kinergetics
Philip Rafferty, 88 Emu Bay Rd, Deloraine, Tasmania 7304, Australia
Phone: 03 6362 2657
philip.rafferty@gmail.com
www.reset-tmj.com
www.kinergetics.com.au

The Kinesiology Academy
registrar@kinesiologyacademy.com.au
www.kinesiologyacademy.com.au

Kinesiology: An Application for Professionals
113 Eyre Street, Seaview Downs, South Australia 5049, Australia
Phone: 403 815 622
ammann@dynamickinesiology.com
www.dyanmickinesiology.com

Neuro-Training P/L
100 Magellan St, First Floor, Lismore, NSW 2480, Australia
Phone: 02 66221514
info@neuro-training.com
www.neuro-training.com

Sips Kinesiology Pty Ltd
21 Maroong Drive, Research, Victoria 3095, Australia
Phone: 03 9437 2495
Sipskinesiology@bigpond.com

Touch for Health Instructors Association of Australia
email@touch4health.org.au
www.touch4health.org.au

Belgium

Institut Belge de Kinesiologie, IBK
avenue Paul Nicodème, 26, 1330 Rixensart, Belgium
www.ibk.be

Fédération Belge de Kinésiologie
Rue Herman, 14, 1315 Incourt, Belgium
info@kinesiology-belgium.org
www.kinesiology-belgium.org

Canada

Canadian Association of Specialized Kinesiology (CanASK)
Box 45071, Vancouver, British Columbia, V3S 2M8, Canada
Phone: 604 669 8481
office@canask.org
www.canask.org

Canadian Kinesiology Bookstore
483 Glenholme Street, Coquitlam, BC, V3K 5E1 Canada
Phone: 604 936 5463
orders@kinesiologybooks.net
www.kinesiologybooks.net

Health Kinesiology Inc
1304 Asphodel Line 2, RR3 Hastings, K0L 1Y0, Canada
Phone: 705 696 3176
hk.office@hk-training.org
www.subtlenergy.com
www.HK-Training.org
www.HK-Practitioners.net
www.hk4health.co.uk

Denmark
Dansk Pædagogisk Kinesiologiskole
www.kinesiologiuddannelse.dk

Polaris International College (Transformational Kinesiology)
Kyndeløse Strandvej 22, DK-4070 Kirke Hyllinge, Denmark
Tel: 46 4066 50
adm@polariscentret.dk
www.polarisdk.dk

Finland
Finnish Kinesiology Association
Suomen kinesiolgiayhdistys ry, Pelimannintie 13 A, 00420 Helsinki, Finland
Phone:3 58 9 - 4789 2189, 358 40 - 821 7115
kinesiologiayhdistys@kaapeli.fi
www.kinesiologia.fi

France
IFKA (Institut Français de Kinésiologie Appliquée)
6 rue Barginet, 38000 Grenoble, France
Phone: 09 88 77 50 90
info@ifka.com
www.ifka.com

Germany
Akademie für Kinesiologie und Heilkunde
Englitzweg 15, D-88147 Achberg / Bodensee, Germany
www.integrative.de

Bio-Energetic Tools & More (online kinesiology store)
Germany
Phone: 07836 957 9911
bio-tools@seminarhaus-krone.com

Deutsche Ärztegesellschaft für Applied Kinesiology (DÄGAK)
Nederlinger Str. 35, D-80638 München, Germany
Phone: 0 89-1595951
DAEGAKPAKinD@aol.com
www.DAEGAK.de

Deutsche Gesellschaft für Angewandte Kinesiologie, DGAK
Dietenbacherstr. 22, 79199 Kirchzarten, Germany
www.dgak.de

Gabriele Schäfer-Matthies und Klaus Schäfer (Health Kinesiology)
79227 Schallstadt, Germany
Phone 07664 618118
www.kschaefer.de
www.schaefer-matthies.de

IAK Institut für Angewandte Kinesiologie GmbH
Eschbachstr. 5, 79199 Kirchzarten bei Freiburg, Germany
Phone: 0 76 61 / 98 71 0
www.iak-freiburg.de
info@iak-freiburg.de

Internationale Kinesiologie Akademie
Cunostr. 50-52, 60388 Frankfurt am Main, Germany
Phone: 061 09 - 72 39 41
info@kinesiologie-akademie.de
www.kinesiologie-akademie.de

VAK Verlags GmbH (kinesiology online shop and publisher)
Eschbachstraße 5, 79199 Kirchzarten, Germany
Phone: 07661-9871-50
info@vakverlag.de
www.vakverlag.de

Vibrana - Schäfer und Matthies GbR (kinesiology online shop)
79227 Schallstadt, Germany
Phone 07664 617277
www.vibrana.de

Ireland

Association of Systematic Kinesiology In Ireland (ASK Ireland)
Roe Kilmeena, Westport, Co Mayo, Ireland
support@kinesiology.ie
www.kinesiology.ie

Harmony Holistics Kinesiology College
Nenagh, Co Tipperary Ireland
086 823 7714
www.harmonyholistics.com
info@harmonyholistics.com

Kinesiology College of Ireland
1 Rockgrove, Midleton, Co. Cork, Ireland
021 4633421
ger@kinesiologycollege.com
www.kinesiologycollege.com

Italy

Accademia di Kinesiologia
Via Rutilia 22, 20141 Milano, Italy
Tel: 02533634
info@accademiadikinesiologia.it
www.accademiadikinesiologia.it

Federazione di Kinesiologia (Italy)
info@federazionedikinesiologia.org
www.federazionedikinesiologia.org

Japan

Japan Kinesiology Institute
zenkinesiology@gmail.com

Japan Touch for Health Kinesiology Association
touch4health@kinesiology.jp

Kineseedlight
J-plaza 4F, 2-99 Motomachi, Naka-ku, Yokohama, Japan 231-0861
Phone: 045 662 1456
www.kinesiology.co.jp
www.kinesiology-seminar.com

Mexico

Centro Integral de Kinesiología Aplicada
Guerrero 94, Col. Del Carmen, Coyoacán, 04100, D. F., México
info@cika.com.mx
www.cika.com.mx

New Zealand
Australasian College of Kinesiology Mastery
info@ackm.edu.au
www.ackm.edu.au or www.kinesiology.edu.au

Kinesiology Association of New Zealand
www.kanz.co.nz

Norway
Den Norske Kinesiologforening (The Norwegian Kinesiology Association)
Postboks 195, Mangleru, 0612 Oslo, Norway
0954 37 751
sekretar@dnkf.org
www.dnkf.org

South Africa
Association of Specialised Kinesiologists South Africa
www.kinesiologysa.co.za

Spain
Vida kinesiologia
c/ onze de setembre 9 -11 passatge, 08160 Montmelo, Spain
Phone: 935684024
vida@vidakine.com
www.vidakine.com

Sweden
Kinesiologer
www.kinesiologer.se

Svenska Kinesiologiskolan
www.kinesiologi.se

Switzerland
Berner Institut für Kinesiologie BIK
Seftigenstrasse 41, 3007 Bern, Switzerland
kinesiologie@bik.ch
www.bik.ch

Schweizerischer Verband Nicht-Medizinische Kinesiologie
Association Suisse pour la Kinésiologie non médicale
Associazione Svizzera della Kinesiologia non medicinale
www.svnmk.ch

United Kingdom

Association of Systematic Kinesiology (ASK)
104a Sedlescombe Road North, St Leonards on Sea, East Sussex TN37 7EN, UK
Phone: 0845 0200383
admin@systematic-kinesiology.co.uk
www.systematic-kinesiology.co.uk

Classical Kinesiology Institute
81, Lancashire Street, Leicester, LE4 7AF, UK
Phone: 0116 266 1962
info@classicalkinesiology.co.uk
www.classicalkinesiology.co.uk

Creative Kinesiology
10 Forestry Houses, Bellever, Postbridge, Devon PL20 6TP, UK
Phone: 01822 880264
info@creativekinesiology.org
www.creativekinesiology.org
www.lifetracking.net

Harmony College
575 Anniesland Road, Scotstounhill, Glasgow, G13 1UX, Scotland
Phone: 0141 954 1796
www.harmonykinesiology.com

Health Kinesiology
08707 655980
info@hk4health.co.uk
www.hk4health.co.uk

Kinesiology Federation (UK)
PO Box 28908, Dalkeith, EH22 2YQ, Scotland
Phone: 0845 260 1094
admin@kinesiologyfederation.co.uk
www.kinesiologyfederation.co.uk

Life-Work Potential Limited (kinesiology online shop)
www.lifeworkpotential.com

Optimum Health Balance
23 Church Lane, Burgh-next-Aylsham, Norwich, NR11 6TR, UK
Phone: 01263 732197
gill@kinesiologyohb.co.uk
www.kinesiologyohb.co.uk

Progressive Kinesiology Academy
10 Barn Fields, Stanway, Colchester, Essex, CO3 0WL, UK
Phone: 01206 570143
info@progressive-kinesiology.co.uk
www.progressive-kinesiology.co.uk

Touch for Health (UK)
www.touchforhealthkinesiology.co.uk
www.kinesiologytraining.co.uk

USA

American College of NeuroEnergetic Kinesiology
8817 So. Redwood Rd, #C, West Jordan, Utah 84088, USA
Phone: 801-566-6262 - USA
ron@acnek.com
www.acnek.com

Applied Physiology
3014 E. Michigan Street, Tucson, AZ 85714, USA
Phone 520-573-3743
iiap@appliedphysiology.com
www.appliedphysiology.com

Crossinology® Brain Integration Technique
Learning Enhancement Center
3704 North 26th Street
Boulder, Colorado 80304, USA
Phone: 303 449 1969
lecboulder@aol.com
www.crossinology.com

Energy Kinesiology Association — EnKA®
11322 Golf Round Dr, New Port Richey, FL 34654, USA
Phone: 866-365-4336
info@energyk.org
www.energyk.org

Institute Of Bioenergetic Arts & Sciences
adam@kinesiohealth.com
www.kinesiohealth.com/html/Programs/AP/aphome.html

The Kinesiology Institute
4712 Admiralty Way, Ste.204, Marina Del Rey, CA 90292, USA
Phone: 800 501 4878
www.kinesiologyinstitute.com

Touch for Health Kinesiology Association
7121 New Light Trail, Chapel Hill, NC, 27516, USA
Phone: 919-969-0027
admin@TFHKA.org
www.TFHKA.org

U.S. Kinesiology Training Institute
7121 New Light Trail, Chapel Hill, NC 27516, USA
greentfh@mindspring.com
www.uskinesiology.com

Lightning Source UK Ltd.
Milton Keynes UK
08 April 2011